Unveiling the Invisible: A Guide to Managing Fibromyalgia

Dedication

To my two beautiful children, Maro and George.

To all patients with fibromyalgia

Acknowledgement

To Linda Kollenburg and Dr Erkan Kurt for designing the book cover.

All rights are preserved for the publisher, The MG Academy LLC. No part of this book may be reproduced or transmitted in any form or by any means, electronic or mechanical, including photocopying, recording, or by any information storage and retrieval system without permission in writing from the copyright owner, The MG Academy LLC.

First edition: 2024.
ISBN: 9798301076169

Table of Contents

Chapter 1—Introduction	1
Chapter 2—Fibromyalgia: Symptoms, Signs, and Diagnosis	5
Chapter 3—Pathophysiology of Fibromyalgia	30
Chapter 4—Risk Factors of Fibromyalgia	43
Chapter 5—Non-Pharmacological Management of Fibromyalgia	58
Chapter 6—Nutrition and Fibromyalgia	86
Chapter 7—Psychological Support and Coping	110
Chapter 8—Medication Management for Fibromyalgia	130
Chapter 9—Role of Interventional Pain	149

Preface

Chronic pain is a pervasive and debilitating condition that affects millions worldwide, with fibromyalgia standing out as a particularly complex disorder. Characterized by widespread musculoskeletal pain, fatigue, sleep disturbances, and heightened sensitivity to pain, fibromyalgia remains a challenging condition for both patients and healthcare providers. While the origins of fibromyalgia are not fully understood, emerging research suggests a malfunction in the central nervous system, causing amplified pain signals throughout the body. As a result, patients with fibromyalgia often endure persistent discomfort, significantly impacting their quality of life.

The treatment of fibromyalgia has traditionally relied on pharmacological therapies, in recent years, interventional pain management techniques have gained prominence, offering novel and effective options for patients suffering from chronic pain, including fibromyalgia.

This book aims to provide an updated and comprehensive guide to these advancements, empowering clinicians to consider new avenues in the management of fibromyalgia and chronic pain. However, pain is rarely a purely physical phenomenon—it often intertwines with psychological, social, and behavioral factors. Recognizing this, this book also emphasizes a holistic approach to pain management. Chapters explore the integration of psychosocial interventions, cognitive-behavioral therapy, mindfulness practices, and mental health support in addressing the multifaceted nature of chronic pain. By focusing on the physical and emotional dimensions of pain, this book underscores the importance of treating the whole person, not just the symptoms.

As multiple authors contribute to this work, the perspectives shared reflect a collective commitment to advancing the field of pain management and providing better care for patients suffering from fibromyalgia. The insights and evidence presented will inspire further research, clinical application, and, ultimately, improved outcomes for individuals living with this challenging condition.

Alaa Abd-Elsayed, MD, MBA, MPH, CPE, FASA

Introduction

Alaa Abd-Elsayed

Fibromyalgia is a complex and often misunderstood chronic pain disorder, one that continues to pose significant challenges to patients and healthcare professionals alike. Despite significant advancements in medical technology and research, the etiology of fibromyalgia remains elusive, complicating both diagnosis and treatment. Chronic pain, as a broad diagnosis, affects an estimated 20% of the global population, making it a critical area of concern in modern medicine. Among these, fibromyalgia stands out as a particularly perplexing condition. It is estimated that 2.7% of the global population suffers from fibromyalgia, with prevalence rates in the United States reaching as high as 6.4%. This rise in diagnoses underscores the immense personal and societal burden of fibromyalgia, which has become a global public health issue.

Fibromyalgia is most often linked to widespread muscle and joint pain, but its effects go far beyond physical discomfort. People with fibromyalgia may also experience problems with memory and concentration, emotional distress, and a variety of other symptoms that affect their overall well-being. Because the condition presents with such a wide range of symptoms, it can be challenging to diagnose and even harder to treat. Many patients spend years searching for answers, feeling frustrated as they navigate the healthcare system. Although the disorder was first mentioned in medical writings as early as 1592, our understanding of fibromyalgia has evolved. The term "fibromyalgia" itself was introduced in 1976, but earlier references show that the struggle to understand the condition has been ongoing for centuries.

The journey to diagnosis is often long and filled with uncertainty. Patients frequently see multiple healthcare providers, including rheumatologists, neurologists, psychiatrists, and pain specialists, before receiving a definitive diagnosis. This process can lead to emotional and physical exhaustion, as well as increased healthcare utilization and costs. A multidisciplinary approach to care is essential for improving outcomes, but without it, patients risk inadequate care that exacerbates the challenges of living with fibromyalgia. Specialized care teams—including rheumatologists, neurologists, chronic pain specialists, and mental health professionals—are necessary to address the multifaceted nature of the disease, offering tailored interventions that target not only the physical pain but also the psychological and cognitive symptoms that accompany it.

Fibromyalgia is more prevalent in women than in men, with the disparity in prevalence rates sparking ongoing research into potential hormonal, genetic, and environmental factors that may contribute to its development. While fibromyalgia can occur at any age, it most commonly manifests after the age of 30, with peak incidence occurring between 40 and 60 years. Yet, the condition's reach extends beyond adults, with juvenile fibromyalgia being a recognized subset that further complicates the disease's profile.

The growing prevalence of fibromyalgia demands improved diagnostic tools, better treatment options, and a clearer understanding of its pathophysiology. Healthcare providers across all specialties must be equipped to care for fibromyalgia patients, especially in perioperative settings, where pain management and anesthesia present unique challenges. As the burden of fibromyalgia increases, healthcare systems must adapt to meet the ongoing needs of patients who suffer from chronic pain, fatigue, and cognitive dysfunction, often without a definitive diagnosis.

This book aims to provide a comprehensive exploration of fibromyalgia, from its historical origins to its current diagnostic criteria, and to delve into the symptoms, treatment modalities, and multidisciplinary approaches that are essential for improving patient outcomes. Through a deeper understanding of this complex disorder, we hope to foster greater empathy, awareness, and collaboration among healthcare providers, ensuring that fibromyalgia patients receive the care and support they need to lead fulfilling lives despite the challenges they face.

In the chapters that follow, we will examine the various facets of fibromyalgia, including the latest research on its pathophysiology, the evolving diagnostic criteria, and the array of treatment options available. With a focus on patient-centered care, this book emphasizes the importance of a holistic approach that considers not only the physical aspects of fibromyalgia but also its psychological, cognitive, and social implications. By broadening the scope of our understanding, we can better address the complex needs of fibromyalgia patients and contribute to the growing body of knowledge that will ultimately lead to improved diagnosis, treatment, and quality of life for those affected.

Fibromyalgia: Symptoms, Signs, and Diagnosis

Hanna Marie William

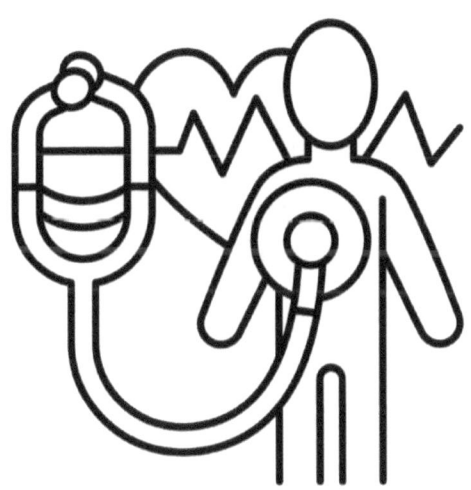

Fibromyalgia is a complex chronic pain disorder with complexities spanning across signs, symptoms, and diagnosis. Although there has been much development in technology, which has contributed to significant research and advancements in medicine, the condition's etiology remains unclear. Chronic pain as a broad diagnosis is very common, with studies showing that it affects about 20% of the world's population. This statistic is quite alarming and demands a consideration of the massive challenges presented by fibromyalgia and other chronic pain disorders. These conditions place a heavy burden on individuals and healthcare systems internationally[1]. Studies estimate that fibromyalgia affects 2.7% of the global population and that the prevalence rates in the United States are estimated at around 6.4%[23]. This shows a tremendous growth trend over the years, demonstrating that the burden of fibromyalgia is significant across the globe.

Fibromyalgia is most commonly associated with chronic pain, frequently musculoskeletal; this can affect many parts of the body. The vague symptomatology of fibromyalgia can make the condition challenging to diagnose and subsequently manage effectively.

The term "fibromyalgia" was first used in 1976 to describe a specific type of rheumatism that does not involve joint inflammation; this distinguished the condition from other rheumatic disease types[3]. Although the term "fibromyalgia" was not used before 1976, the history of fibromyalgia extends much further back. Early medical practitioners and scientists used several other terms to describe what we now understand to be fibromyalgia symptoms. As early as 1592, most people used the term "muscular rheumatism" to refer to the condition. Then, in

1904, the term "fibrositis" became common as a way to describe the inflammation of fibrous tissue in the body, which was thought to be the root cause of the disorder at the time. Later on, in 1941, the term "rheumatic myalgia" described the common muscular pain linked with the condition. Notably, this basic history demonstrates how our understanding of fibromyalgia has changed over time and hints at the complexities involved in recognizing its signs, symptoms, and diagnosis.

A multidisciplinary approach is critical for the management of fibromyalgia. It should be the standard of care to consider the expertise of numerous diverse medical specialists for the benefit of fibromyalgia patients. Understandably, the lack of multidisciplinary involvement can lead to inadequate care, frustration, and increased burden on patients and their families. Rheumatologists, who specialize in diseases of the musculoskeletal system and various autoimmune disorders, often take the lead in diagnosing and treating fibromyalgia. Neurologists play an important role in managing neurologic components of the disease, such as cognitive dysfunction and central sensitization (a phenomenon that occurs when the central nervous system's response to pain is amplified, leading to hypersensitivity to pain or hyperalgesia)[15,26]. Chronic pain specialists are also valuable on the treatment team, as they can offer multi-modal pain management strategies tailored to the needs of individual fibromyalgia patients.

Finally, psychiatrists are sometimes involved in the care of these patients to address neuropsychiatric symptoms, such as anxiety, depression, and sleep disorders, which frequently accompany fibromyalgia[3].

Epidemiologic data has shown that fibromyalgia is more prevalent among women than among men, with an estimated prevalence of 7.7% in women compared to 4.9% in men[3]. Such gender disparity has been the subject of much research, with theories suggesting that hormonal, genetic, or social factors may contribute to the higher prevalence of fibromyalgia in women[34]. Additionally, although fibromyalgia can be diagnosed at any age, it tends to be more common after the age of 30[4,5,6]. There are suggestions that fibromyalgia incidence increases with age and peaks in individuals between the ages of 40 and 60. However, there are certainly cases where younger patients, including children and adolescents, are diagnosed with fibromyalgia, further emphasizing the variable nature of this condition[28]. There is even a subset of fibromyalgia known as juvenile-onset fibromyalgia[28,29].

The prevalence of fibromyalgia is constantly rising, making it crucial to better understand the various aspects that can improve interventions and healthcare capabilities to address it. Healthcare providers across all medical specialties will almost certainly encounter patients with fibromyalgia at some point in their careers. Consequently, physicians must have a thorough understanding of the disease to provide optimal care to their patients. For example, anesthesia and surgery providers caring for fibromyalgia patients in the perioperative setting should be aware of the unique complexities that the disorder contributes to their care. Anesthesia and surgery providers should know that patients with fibromyalgia often have heightened sensitivity to pain, which can complicate pain management during and after surgery[15]. This feature necessitates additional management considerations to ensure that patients with fibromyalgia receive appropriate and effective acute pain relief in the perioperative setting and beyond.

With the rising of fibromyalgia diagnoses almost everywhere across the globe, the condition is becoming more and more of a significant public health concern[3]. Patients with fibromyalgia face chronic struggles, often dealing with persistent pain, fatigue, and cognitive difficulties for years before having a named diagnosis. Many of the patients inadvertently end up seeing multiple healthcare providers, including specialists in rheumatology, neurology, and psychiatry, over the years in search of a diagnosis and effective treatment[3,8]. They often try several different treatment modalities, including medications, physical therapy, cognitive behavioral therapy, and other alternative therapies, such as acupuncture and massage therapies. Unfortunately, the effectiveness of these treatments can vary greatly from patient to patient, making it difficult to find a consistent and successful management strategy to recommend to patients across the board.

Fibromyalgia increases healthcare utilization in general while also contributing to raised healthcare costs for patients individually. One of the biggest contributors to this high cost of healthcare stems from the fact that individuals with fibromyalgia attend nearly twice as many healthcare appointments as patients without this condition[3,7]. According to research, fibromyalgia patients incur healthcare costs that are approximately three times higher than those of the general population[7]. These remarkable statistics are also likely influenced by the condition being so complex and demanding in terms of the need for long-term, ongoing care from multiple specialists and as well as frequent adjustments to treatment plans. The economic burden of fibromyalgia is further compounded by barriers to accessing appropriate healthcare, which further contributes to reduced quality of life for these patients[27]. Many fibromyalgia patients report difficulties finding healthcare providers who are knowledgeable about their condition or who take their symptoms seriously[30]. These patients can easily get ignored and their symptoms written off. The barriers can delay diagnosis and treatment, leading to worse outcomes for patients and increased healthcare costs over time.

It is crucial to encourage and support new and advanced research focusing on fibromyalgia to improve the understanding of the disease and its pathophysiology. Getting a better understanding of the disease's pathophysiology and etiology could easily inform the development of more effective treatments. Subsequently, healthcare providers must work collaboratively across specialties to support patients with fibromyalgia, offering them a comprehensive range of treatments and resources. This chapter will provide an overview of the symptoms, signs, and diagnosis of fibromyalgia.

Symptoms and Signs

Fibromyalgia symptoms usually involve multiple organ systems, which contribute to the condition's well-known complexity, especially when it comes to diagnosis and management. Notably, the broad symptomatology often leads to diagnostic challenges because the condition can mimic or overlap with various other disorders. The variability in how fibromyalgia manifests among individuals, paired with an incomplete understanding of its pathophysiology, makes the condition even more difficult for both patients and healthcare providers to manage[7]. Several theories have been proposed to explain the diverse and widespread symptoms of fibromyalgia. Generally speaking, fibromyalgia involves some issues with the central nervous system's processing of pain signals[9]. As previously mentioned, it leads to a heightened sensitivity to pain, also known as central sensitization[9]. The dysfunction in pain processing is thought to be a key mechanism in the manifestation of fibromyalgia, although it is likely not the only factor involved.

According to studies focused on understanding the risk factors for fibromyalgia, it is not abundantly clear, but the disorder might run in families or have a potential genetic component. Consequently, certain genetic variations could increase susceptibility to developing the condition[10]. Environmental factors, such as infections, physical trauma, and significant emotional stress, are also thought to act as potential triggers for the onset of fibromyalgia in genetically predisposed individuals[16,17,18]. Although it is unknown to what extent environmental versus genetic factors play a role in fibromyalgia, the two factors are crucial in contributing to its onset.

Widespread musculoskeletal pain is the hallmark symptom of fibromyalgia that comes to mind for most people. This often affects both sides of the body and spans across both the upper and lower extremities. In terms of intensity, the pain can range from mild discomfort to severe and acute pain, which is the more common debilitating symptom that interferes with daily activities[12]. Some patients report fluctuations in the severity of their pain and migrations of the pain's location throughout their lives and the course of the disease. Additionally, fibromyalgia patients often experience pain in response to stimuli that would not normally be considered painful, which is known as allodynia. This heightened pain response can make even routine activities, such as light touch or wearing certain clothing, uncomfortable or painful.

The disruption in central nervous system sensation is not limited to pain; some fibromyalgia patients report alternative sensory disturbances such as paresthesia. These could include sensations of tingling, numbness, or burning in the extremities.[13] The symptoms can be distressing or even make the diagnosis more complicated. Because paresthesia is a common symptom in other neurological conditions (stroke, nerve entrapment, multiple sclerosis, diabetic neuropathy, etc.), this symptom can cloud a patient's clinical picture and contribute to difficulty in diagnosis. Headaches, including tension headaches and migraines, are also commonly reported among fibromyalgia patients and can significantly contribute to the overall burden of the disease[13].

The chronicity of the condition's symptoms often leads to other secondary symptoms, including psychological and cognitive issues. Many patients eventually become hypervigilant to pain, feeling constantly on high alert for potential triggers or flare-ups of their symptoms. When combined with other symptoms, as well as the financial and societal burdens of fibromyalgia, hypervigilance can contribute to further emotional distress and mental fatigue. As a result, some individuals with fibromyalgia develop mood disorders such as anxiety and depression. It is estimated that 30-50% of fibromyalgia patients have a concurrent diagnosis of anxiety or depression at the time of their diagnosis[9,11]. The psychological symptoms may then exacerbate the perception of pain, creating a vicious cycle that further impacts the patient's quality of life.

Besides mood disturbances, cognitive symptoms are also quite common in fibromyalgia. The cognitive symptoms are sometimes referred to as "fibro fog"[31]. Patients report difficulties with memory, concentration, and overall mental clarity. Consequently, it can make even simple tasks feel overwhelming. Although not physically debilitating, the cognitive impairment aspect can be as distressing and disruptive to everyday life as the physical symptoms of pain and fatigue. Patients experiencing "fibro fog" often struggle to function at work or even to manage daily responsibilities and tasks. The symptoms can sometimes wax and wane or even correlate with the other physical symptoms of fibromyalgia. They can worsen during periods of heightened pain or stress, which is often a distressing experience for patients.

Fibromyalgia is also frequently associated with gastrointestinal issues. Concurrence of fibromyalgia with irritable bowel syndrome (IBS) and gastroesophageal reflux disease (GERD) are particularly common[9]. These gastrointestinal conditions can cause abdominal pain, bloating, diarrhea, constipation, and acid reflux, all of which add yet another layer of complexity to the symptom profile of fibromyalgia. The relationship between fibromyalgia and gastrointestinal dysfunction is not fully understood, but it has been suggested that both conditions may share common pathophysiological mechanisms, particularly involving the autonomic nervous system[9].

Furthermore, many fibromyalgia patients experience a wide range of other systemic complaints. For example, dry eyes and dry mouth are commonly reported, which may also be related to dysregulation of the autonomic nervous system[14]. Some patients have trouble breathing (dyspnea) without an identifiable respiratory cause, and others struggle with dysphagia or difficulty swallowing, which can further complicate the management of their symptoms[14]. Malnutrition can become an issue for these patients as well. Palpitations, or irregular heartbeats, are another symptom that some patients experience, although these are typically benign and usually not associated with an underlying cardiovascular pathology[32]. The presence of these varied symptoms often leads to extensive testing and specialist consultations as healthcare providers work to rule out other potential causes before formally diagnosing fibromyalgia.

Fibromyalgia's multiple symptoms across multiple organ systems with often unclear relationships make the diagnosis complicated and make it difficult for clinicians to recognize it, especially in its early stages. Ultimately, complex patient presentations commonly result in delayed diagnosis and subsequent treatment. Oftentimes, patients have to see multiple healthcare providers and undergo numerous tests before a diagnosis can be made. Clinicians have to remain vigilant in considering fibromyalgia as a diagnosis when faced with a patient who presents with widespread pain and a constellation of other seemingly unrelated symptoms.

There are only a few signs that clinicians can identify or even associate with fibromyalgia during a standardized physical examination. Fibromyalgia does not cause the visible joint swelling or deformities seen in other rheumatological conditions. Nevertheless, the patients may exhibit tenderness to palpation at specific points on the body, known as tender points[33]. Although the tender points were once a central feature of fibromyalgia diagnosis, they are now considered only one aspect of a broader diagnostic picture. The relative absence of physical exam findings or other visible signs of inflammation, combined with the presence of widespread pain and associated symptoms, can help guide clinicians toward a diagnosis of fibromyalgia.

Diagnosis

There has been a significant growth in the attempts to establish standardized diagnostic criteria for fibromyalgia. However, many have been somewhat controversial and have sparked debate. There was decent criticism of early diagnostic efforts in fibromyalgia diagnosis, especially due to the incompleteness of these diagnostic tools, which were found by many to be significantly limited in scope or overall diagnostic value. In 1990, the American College of Rheumatology (ACR) introduced one of the more significant and successful attempts at establishing a framework for the diagnosis of fibromyalgia. This framework outlined specific diagnostic criteria for fibromyalgia for the first time[9].

The ACR criteria focused on identifying tenderness to pressure or palpation at 11 out of 18 defined points on the body, referred to as "tender points."[9] The 18 defined points are specific anatomical locations, including the base of the neck, upper chest, shoulders, hips, and knees, where fibromyalgia patients typically experience heightened sensitivity and pain with even light pressure[9].

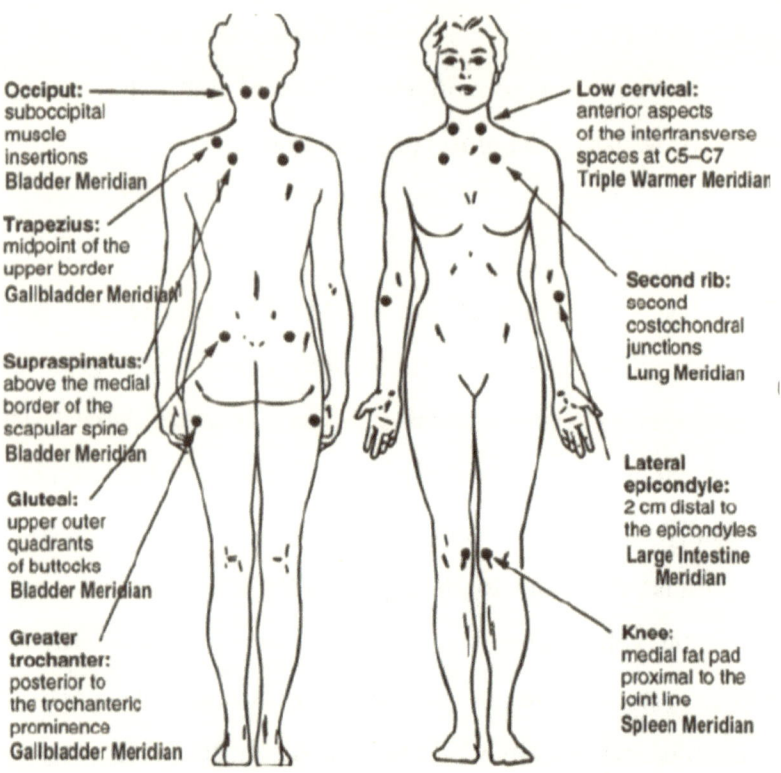

Although the specific diagnostic criteria have since changed, the initial establishment of a detailed framework for the diagnosis of fibromyalgia was significant in equipping healthcare professionals with the tools needed to identify and acknowledge patients who are struggling with this condition. Having official diagnostic criteria from a professional medical organization assists in the overall validation that fibromyalgia is a medical condition that should be given serious diagnostic and therapeutic consideration.

Despite being a massive step towards improved recognition of fibromyalgia as a legitimate medical condition, the 1990 criteria were massively limited in so many aspects. One of the main issues with this approach was the difficulty physicians faced in accurately and consistently assessing the so-called tender points. The examination to assess tender points as described relied heavily on a provider's subjective judgment, which then led to high variability in diagnosis depending on the clinician's experience, technique, and opinion. It also left the door open for biases about fibromyalgia as an overall condition, the specific patient population that is affected by the condition, and the concept of pain in general to influence diagnosis. The examination suggested by this criteria disregarded non-musculoskeletal symptoms such as cognitive difficulties, fatigue, and psychological disturbances, which are now known to be core components of the disorder[9]. The shortcomings contributed to widespread dissatisfaction with the initial criteria. A need for improvement in the diagnostic framework prompted the ACR to introduce new criteria in 2010; these were further refined in 2011 and 2016[9]. The updates broadened the scope of fibromyalgia diagnosis. Instead of strictly relying on tender points, a more holistic approach that considered the wide range of symptoms that fibromyalgia patients experience was taken. According to the more recent criteria, fibromyalgia diagnostic criteria are based on three key components: first, the patient must have a Widespread Pain Index (WPI) score of at least 7 out of 19 areas; second, their symptoms must have been present for at least three months with a consistent level of severity (as confirmed by the Symptom Severity Score (SSS)); and third, no other medical condition should explain their symptoms better[9]. By including the WPI and the Symptom Severity Score (SSS) in these new criteria, the medical field as a whole took a huge step towards a much improved diagnostic tool for fibromyalgia, ultimately offering a more symptom-centered and, importantly, objective approach.

As a scoring system, the Widespread Pain Index assesses the number of distinct body regions out of a defined list of 19 areas where a patient has experienced pain over the past week. Example areas are the right and left jaw, shoulder girdles, upper and lower arms, hips, legs, back, neck, chest, and abdomen[19]. Each area where pain is reported contributes to the WPI score. In parallel, the Symptom Severity Score quantifies the subjective severity of common fibromyalgia symptoms, including non-musculoskeletal symptoms such as fatigue, sleep disturbances, and cognitive problems. The SSS is reported per symptom on a scale of 0 to 3, with a total possible score of 12. An SSS score of 0 indicates no significant symptoms, while a score of 3 signifies severe, persistent symptoms that disrupt daily activities. To meet the diagnostic criteria, patients must have a WPI of 7 or more combined with an SSS of at least five or a WPI between 3 and 6 combined with an SSS score of at least 9[20].

The new criteria pay greater attention to symptom diversity, severity, and duration, giving a more comprehensive view of fibromyalgia as a complex condition. Although the diagnostic criteria are a valuable standardized resource, fibromyalgia is largely diagnosed through subjective reports from patients. Consequently, a thorough medical history is essential to rule out other potential causes of the symptoms and to better understand individual patients' symptomatology.

A thorough evaluation with history and physical exam in conjunction with the use of objective diagnostic criteria helps to exclude other disorders that can present with similar symptoms. Some common examples include rheumatoid arthritis, systemic lupus erythematosus,

Sjögren's syndrome, ankylosing spondylitis, polymyalgia rheumatica, inflammatory myositis, irritable bowel syndrome, and chronic headache syndromes like migraines or tension headaches[21]. Part of the diagnostic process could include laboratory testing and imaging. Although there are no proven laboratory markers or imaging findings that confirm the diagnosis, getting this workup can help delineate fibromyalgia from other conditions that may present similarly. Some autoimmune and inflammatory diseases often present with similar symptoms as fibromyalgia but are unique in that they typically cause an elevation in the erythrocyte sedimentation rate (ESR) and C-reactive protein (CRP) labs while fibromyalgia typically does not[21]. Additionally, specific autoantibodies like anti-nuclear antibody (ANA), rheumatoid factor (RF), anti-Smith, anti-double-stranded DNA (dsDNA), and SSA/SSB are frequently elevated in a host of autoimmune or inflammatory diseases but would be normal in patients with fibromyalgia. Other laboratory markers that may be worthwhile in differentiating between fibromyalgia and other conditions with similar symptoms include cyclic citrullinated peptide (CCP) for rheumatoid arthritis, HLA-B27 for ankylosing spondylitis, and serum protein electrophoresis to rule out multiple myeloma or other plasma cell disorders[23]. These tests are tools that clinicians use to exclude other diagnoses and narrow the differential diagnosis when considering fibromyalgia as a diagnosis. They do not confirm the diagnosis of fibromyalgia but rather exclusion of other diagnoses. Notably, their significance is massively expounded when symptoms overlap or are vague.

It is also clear that certain imaging studies can be useful to evaluate patients presenting with symptoms concerning fibromyalgia.

As mentioned previously, fibromyalgia symptoms include widespread pain. It is important to ensure that careful attention is paid to areas of pain and that these areas are evaluated properly. There may be injuries or other diagnoses contributing to pain that can be diagnosed with imaging. Most commonly, the imaging modalities used to investigate are CT and MRI imaging. A herniated disc can be highlighted through the use of imaging studies and could be the cause of a patient's back pain, while rheumatoid arthritis may explain another patient's joint pain after imaging findings suggest this diagnosis. There is typically no visual finding on imaging that correlates to symptoms in patients with fibromyalgia. Imaging studies in these cases are usually unremarkable as the pain does not directly result from a physical pathology but instead from altered processing of pain, as discussed previously[24].

Labs and imaging do not play a diagnostic role in fibromyalgia. This has been somewhat frustrating to medical professionals and patients alike as it makes the condition difficult to diagnose. It will be helpful to have future studies focusing on understanding the biomarkers that may be associated with fibromyalgia to alleviate some of the challenges in diagnosing the condition. Although there have been numerous studies attempting to find a biological marker of the disorder, none have proven reliable in clinical practice. Prior research had suggested that an antibody called antipolymer may be the biomarker that researchers have been looking for to aid in the diagnosis of fibromyalgia. Further investigation, unfortunately, determined that antipolymer was only present in 17.6% of fibromyalgia patients, making it an inadequate marker to use for diagnosis[23]. Other studies have suggested anti-serotonin, antiganglioside, and antiphospholipid antibodies as being diagnostically significant in fibromyalgia patients.

None of these markers have been adopted as diagnostic tools because they are not sensitive enough[24]. Further research is needed to find a biomarker that is specific enough to be used diagnostically. Finding a laboratory test that would reliably suggest a diagnosis of fibromyalgia would aid in making this difficult diagnosis more straightforward and objective. It would be correct to consider fibromyalgia a diagnosis of exclusion, especially for the lack of suggestive laboratory or imaging findings and with most symptoms overlapping with other conditions. A good history and physical exam, along with the ACS criteria, can help guide the road to diagnosis for providers and their patients. An open-minded provider who listens to their patient's history is the most valuable diagnostic tool. With its complexity and broad symptomatology, providers must carefully evaluate each patient and adequately rule out another diagnosis as they are able before confirming a diagnosis of fibromyalgia. The diagnosis relies heavily on clinical judgment. As research into fibromyalgia continues to advance, we hope that new diagnostic techniques become available and are implemented for the benefit of fibromyalgia patients. More reliable, concrete, objective, and unbiased diagnostic approaches will improve care for these patients and help alleviate at least one frustrating aspect of their struggle with this debilitating condition.

Example Case
The patient is a 45-year-old woman with a history of depression, gastroesophageal reflux disease, and hypertension who presents to her primary care physician with a six-month history of widespread

musculoskeletal pain and fatigue. She describes the pain as deep and aching that migrates throughout her body and fluctuates in intensity, overall getting worse over the last 4 months. Over this time, the pain has affected her neck, bilateral shoulders, back, and left hip, which she reports are all tender to the touch. Although she sleeps 8 hours per night, she does not feel well rested in the daytime. She also reports feeling brain fog and having difficulty concentrating on daily tasks. The patient denies recent injuries or infections; she denies alcohol or other drug use and only takes omeprazole for reflux symptoms. She reports that her mother had chronic pain but was never formally diagnosed with a condition. Having seen a neurologist and rheumatologist before this presentation, the patient is still without a formal diagnosis of what is contributing to her symptoms.

Physical examination reveals that the patient's vital signs are normal and stable. Her blood pressure is 118/76, her heart rate is 74, and her oxygen saturation is 97% on room air. She appears tired but in no acute distress. She endorses diffuse tenderness to palpation over her trapezius, lower back, chest, and left hip but no swelling or redness. She exhibits tenderness in 11 typical "tender points" for fibromyalgia as defined by the WPI mentioned above. She has been having moderate to severe symptoms in over three areas over the last 4 months, making her SSS score, as defined above, an 8. A full neurological exam shows normal reflexes, strength, and sensation. The patient seems anxious and tearful when discussing her pain, which she acknowledges.

Given her symptoms, a range of conditions are considered, including fibromyalgia, chronic fatigue syndrome, rheumatoid arthritis, lupus, and hypothyroidism. The findings of the laboratory workup are as follows:

- Complete blood count (CBC): Normal.
- Erythrocyte sedimentation rate (ESR) and C-reactive protein (CRP): Both are normal, ruling out significant inflammatory processes.
- Thyroid function tests (TSH, free T4): Normal, which excludes hypothyroidism.
- Rheumatoid factor (RF) and antinuclear antibody (ANA): Negative, making autoimmune conditions like rheumatoid arthritis and lupus less likely.
- Comprehensive metabolic panel (CMP): Normal.
- MRI brain, cervical, thoracic, and lumbar spine: Largely unremarkable besides normal changes expected given age.

The diagnosis of fibromyalgia was made based on the widespread and persistent pain in over seven distinct areas for more than 3 months, fatigue, sleep disturbances, and cognitive complaints, and the lack of abnormal lab results or structural causes to suggest another diagnosis.

References:

1. Goldberg, D.S., McGee, S.J. Pain as a global public health priority. BMC Public Health 11, 770 (2011). https://doi.org/10.1186/1471-2458-11-770
2. Queiroz, L.P. Worldwide Epidemiology of Fibromyalgia. Curr Pain Headache Rep 17, 356 (2013). https://doi.org/10.1007/s11916-013-0356-5
3. Vincent A, Lahr BD, Wolfe F, Clauw DJ, Whipple MO, Oh TH, Barton DL, St Sauver J. Prevalence of fibromyalgia: a population-based study in Olmsted County, Minnesota, utilizing the Rochester Epidemiology Project. Arthritis Care Res (Hoboken). 2013 May;65(5):786-92.
4. McNally J, Matheson D, Bakowsky V. The epidemiology of self-reported fibromyalgia in Canada. Chronic Dis Can. 2006; 27:9–16.
5. Branco J, Bannwarth B, Failde I, et al. Prevalence of fibromyalgia: a survey in five European countries. Semin Arthritis Rheum. 2010; 39:448–53. A large, nationwide epidemiological study of FM in France, Germany, Italy, Portugal, and Spain.
6. Mas A, Carmona L, Valverde M, et al. Prevalence and impact of fibromyalgia on function and quality of life in individuals from the general population: results from a nationwide study in Spain. Clin Exp Reumatol. 2008; 2:519–26.
7. Kocyigit BF, Akyol A. Fibromyalgia syndrome: epidemiology, diagnosis and treatment. Reumatologia. 2022;60(6):413-421. doi: 10.5114/reum.2022.123671. Epub 2022 Dec 30. PMID:

36683836; PMCID: PMC9847104.
8. Marques AP, Santo ASDE, Berssaneti AA, et al. Prevalence of fibromyalgia: literature review update. Rev Bras Reumatol 2017; 57: 356–363, DOI: 10.1016/j.rbre.2017.01.005
9. Bhargava J, Hurley JA. Fibromyalgia. [Updated 2023 Jun 11]. In: StatPearls [Internet]. Treasure Island (FL): StatPearls Publishing; 2024 Jan-. Available from: https://www.ncbi.nlm.nih.gov/books/NBK540974/
10. Markkula R, Järvinen P, Leino-Arjas P, Koskenvuo M, Kalso E, Kaprio J. Clustering of symptoms associated with fibromyalgia in a Finnish Twin Cohort. Eur J Pain 2009; 13:744-50. 10.1016/j.ejpain.2008.09.007
11. Fuller-Thomson E, Nimigon-Young J, Brennenstuhl S. Individuals with fibromyalgia and depression: findings from a nationally representative Canadian survey. Rheumatol Int. 2012 Apr;32(4):853-62.
12. Björkegren K, Wallander MA, Johansson S, Svärdsudd K. General symptom reporting in female fibromyalgia patients and referents: a population-based case-referent study. BMC Public Health. 2009 Oct 31; 9:402.
13. De Tommaso M, Federici A, Serpino C, Vecchio E, Franco G, Sardaro M, Delussi M, Livrea P. Clinical features of headache patients with fibromyalgia comorbidity. J Headache Pain. 2011 Dec;12(6):629-38.
14. Wang JC, Sung FC, Men M, Wang KA, Lin CL, Kao CH. Bidirectional association between fibromyalgia and gastroesophageal reflux disease: two population-based

retrospective cohort analysis. Pain. 2017 Oct;158(10):1971-1978.

15. Maugars Y, Berthelot JM, Le Goff B, Darrieutort-Laffite C. Fibromyalgia and associated disorders: from pain to chronic suffering, from subjective hypersensitivity to hypersensitivity syndrome. Front Med (Lausanne) 2021; 8: 666914, DOI: 10.3389/fmed.2021.666914.

16. Arnold LM, Hudson JI, Hess EV, et al. Family study of fibromyalgia. Arthritis Rheum 2004; 50: 944–952, DOI: 10.1002/art.20042.

17. Clauw DJ. Fibromyalgia: a clinical review. JAMA 2014; 311: 1547–1555, DOI: 10.1001/jama.2014.3266.

18. Sarzi-Puttini P, Giorgi V, Marotto D, Atzeni F. Fibromyalgia: an update on clinical characteristics, etiology and treatment. Nat Rev Rheumatol 2020; 16: 645–660, DOI: 10.1038/s41584-020-00506-w.

19. Dudeney J, Law EF, Meyyappan A, Palermo TM, Rabbitts JA. Evaluating the psychometric properties of the Widespread Pain Index and the Symptom Severity scale in youth with painful conditions. Can J Pain. 2019;3(1):137-147. doi: 10.1080/24740527.2019.1620097. Epub 2019 Jun 26. PMID: 32051925; PMCID: PMC7015535.Arnold LM, Hudson JI, Hess EV, et al. Family study of fibromyalgia. Arthritis Rheum 2004; 50: 944-952, DOI: 10.1002/art.20042.

20. Dizner-Golab A, Lisowska B, Kosson D. Fibromyalgia - etiology, diagnosis and treatment including perioperative management in patients with fibromyalgia. Reumatologia.

2023;61(2):137-148. doi: 10.5114/reum/163094. Epub 2023 May 10. PMID: 37223370; PMCID: PMC10201378.

21. Kaltsas G, Tsiveriotis K. Fibromyalgia. [Updated 2023 Nov 9]. In: Feingold KR, Anawalt B, Blackman MR, et al., editors. Endotext [Internet]. South Dartmouth (MA): MDText.com, Inc.; 2000-. Table 1. [Disorders that can Mimic and/or...]. Available from: https://www.ncbi.nlm.nih.gov/books/NBK279092/table/fibromyalgia.T.disorders_that_can_mimic/

22. Siracusa R, Paola RD, Cuzzocrea S, Impellizzeri D. Fibromyalgia: Pathogenesis, Mechanisms, Diagnosis and Treatment Options Update. International Journal of Molecular Sciences. 2021; 22(8):3891. https://doi.org/10.3390/ijms22083891

23. Iannuccelli, C.; Di Franco, M.; Alessandri, C.; Guzzo, M.P.; Croia, C.; Di Sabato, F.; Foti, M.; Valesini, G. Pathophysiology of fibromyalgia: A comparison with the tension-type headache, a localized pain syndrome. Ann. N. Y. Acad. Sci 2010, 1193, 78–83.

24. Klein, R.; Berg, P.A. High incidence of antibodies to 5-hydroxytryptamine, gangliosides, and phospholipids in patients with chronic fatigue and fibromyalgia syndrome and their relatives: Evidence for a clinical entity of both disorders. Eur. J. Med. Res. 1995, 1, 21–26.

25. Abdulkhaliq A, Alotaibi M. Laboratory Interpretation of Rheumatic Diseases. 2021 Jan 6. In: Almoallim H, Cheikh M, editors. Skills in Rheumatology [Internet]. Singapore: Springer;

2021. Chapter 3. Available from: https://www.ncbi.nlm.nih.gov/books/NBK585756/ doi: 10.1007/978-981-15-8323-0_3

26. Staud, R., Smitherman, M.L. Peripheral and central sensitization in fibromyalgia: Pathogenetic role. Current Science Inc 6, 259–266 (2002). https://doi.org/10.1007/s11916-002-0046-1

27. Marques, A.P., Ferreira, E.A.G., Matsutani, L.A. et al. Quantifying pain threshold and quality of life of fibromyalgia patients. Clin Rheumatol 24, 266–271 (2005). https://doi.org/10.1007/s10067-004-1003-7

28. Coles, M.L., Uziel, Y. Juvenile primary fibromyalgia syndrome: A Review- Treatment and Prognosis. Pediatr Rheumatol 19, 74 (2021). https://doi.org/10.1186/s12969-021-00529-x

29. Kashikar-Zuck S, Cunningham N, Peugh J, et al. Long-term outcomes of adolescents with juvenile-onset fibromyalgia into adulthood and impact of depressive symptoms on functioning over time. Pain. 2019;160(2):433-441. doi: 10.1097/j.pain.0000000000001415

30. Qureshi AG, Jha SK, Iskander J, et al. Diagnostic Challenges and Management of Fibromyalgia. Cureus. 2021;13(10): e18692. Published 2021 Oct 11. doi:10.7759/cureus.18692

31. Dass R, Kalia M, Harris J, Packham T. Understanding the Experience and Impacts of Brain Fog in Chronic Pain: A Scoping Review. Can J Pain. 2023;7(1):2217865. Published

2023 Jul 10. doi:10.1080/24740527.2023.2217865

32. Günlü S, Aktan A. Evaluation of the Cardiac Conduction System in Fibromyalgia Patients With Complaints of Palpitations. Cureus. 2022;14(9): e28784. Published 2022 Sep 5. doi:10.7759/cureus.28784

33. Tunks E, Crook J, Norman G, Kalaher S. Tender points in fibromyalgia. Pain. 1988;34(1):11-19. doi:10.1016/0304-3959(88)90176-5

34. Wolfe F, Walitt B, Perrot S, Rasker JJ, Häuser W. Fibromyalgia diagnosis and biased assessment: Sex, prevalence and bias PLoS One. 2018;13(9):e0203755. Published 2018 Sep

Pathophysiology of Fibromyalgia

George Yacoub

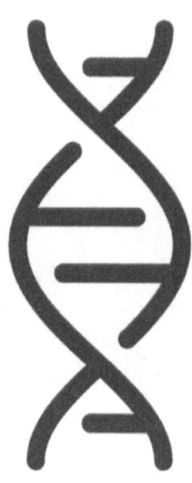

Brain morphology and pain receptors

Fibromyalgia is characterized by central nervous pain dysregulation, as opposed to being a peripheral nerve pathology. This is thought to contribute to the clinical presentation of fibromyalgia as being diffuse or multifocal pain throughout the body rather than pain that localizes to a specific body part or dermatome[1]. This clinical presentation has been termed neoplastic pain by the International Association for the Study of Pain in 2016. This is an important distinction from nociceptive pain, characterized by continuous pain input through tissue damage or inflammation, or neuropathic pain, characterized by peripheral or central nerve damage[2]. The neurophysiology of nociceptive pain is not entirely understood, but an overamplification of central nervous system pain processing pathways is thought to play a major role[3,4]. A meta-analysis review of neuroimaging studies in fibromyalgia published in 2016 notes several brain regions associated with pain that are found to be hyperactive and others that are hypoactive in fibromyalgia patients[5].

Regions noted to be hyperactive in patients with fibromyalgia are the following: the right insula, the primary somatosensory cortex of the left postcentral gyrus, and the right lingual gyrus. The insula plays a role in regulating emotional response to pain and central nervous processing of pain signals from the periphery. The primary somatosensory cortex of the postcentral gyrus has been implicated in the recognition, learning, and memory encoding of painful stimuli. Hyperactivity in this region likely contributes to the impaired perception of pain in the setting of anticipated pain among patients with fibromyalgia[6]. The lingual gyrus plays a role in the analysis of visual information, creativity, emotional self-awareness, and ethical decision-making. Its role in pain perception and modulation is not understood, but studies have shown an association between lingual gyrus activity and pain in patients with migraines and pain anticipation and perception in patients with major depressive disorder[7,8]. Regions noted to be hypoactive in patients with fibromyalgia are the following: the primary somatosensory cortex of the postcentral gyrus, the left anterior cingulate cortex, and the right amygdala. The primary somatosensory cortex of the postcentral gyrus plays a role in the anticipation, quality, intensity, and localization processing of experienced pain. The anterior cingulate cortex and the amygdala both provide inputs to the periaqueductal gray-rostral ventromedial medulla (PAG-RVM) pathway. The PAG-RVM pathway is a descending pathway- from the central nervous system to the peripheral nervous system- that plays a role in inhibiting pain signals in times of stress or when it's disadvantageous to have increased pain sensitivity[9]. Reduced activity in central inhibition of peripheral pain signals like the periaqueductal gray-rostral ventromedial medulla pathway for modulating pain has also long been implicated in the pathophysiology of increased central nervous sensitivity to pain stimuli in fibromyalgia patients[10]. Furthermore, recent studies suggest that fibromyalgia patients have impaired activity in the dorsolateral prefrontal cortex in response to pain stimuli. This brain segment plays a role in modulating and updating pain perception in response to real-time stimuli. Impaired activity in this region suggests that fibromyalgia patients have a reduced capacity to recognize a harmless stimulus and adapt the central processing of the stimulus as being painless when they are anticipating a painful stimulus[11].

Fibromyalgia has also been associated with alterations in central as well as peripheral nervous system morphology. Neuroimaging studies suggest that patients with fibromyalgia have reduced gray matter volume in specific regions of the brain, namely the prefrontal cortex and the anterior cingulate gyrus. These morphological findings correlate with hypoactivity in these brain regions, as discussed in the previous section, and might be a contributing factor to the reduced activity in these regions[12]. Reduced white matter in the left side of the corpus callosum is also associated with fibromyalgia[13]. Although the pathophysiology of these morphological changes is not entirely understood, recent microstructural studies of the brain suggest the role of neuroinflammation in the progression of this disease[14]. Indeed, many studies have previously been performed to assess elevated inflammatory marker levels in the serum and CSF of fibromyalgia patients, but these studies have shown inconsistent findings[15–18]. Aside from the morphological changes, patients with fibromyalgia have a reduced number and density of μ-opioid receptors in several regions of the central nervous system known to play a role in pain modulation, such as the nucleus accumbens, the amygdala, and the dorsal cingulate[19]. This is likely the pathophysiology underlying the lack of efficacy of opioid treatment for patients with fibromyalgia since these treatments target opioid receptors in the central nervous system. In contrast, studies suggest an upregulation and increase of opioid receptors in the skin and periphery of fibromyalgia patients compared to controls. However, the efficacy of applying topical opioids to target peripheral μ-opioid receptors remains to be studied[20,21].

Alterations in neurotransmitter levels

We can also see significant associations between fibromyalgia and the levels of different neurotransmitters involved in the signaling of neuronal pain pathways. Patients with fibromyalgia have been shown to have increased absolute levels of glutamate in the brain cerebrum and cerebrospinal fluid. Glutamate is an excitatory neurotransmitter, and glutamate receptors are involved in multiple pain pathways both in the central and the peripheral nervous system[22,23]. Furthermore, studies show a correlation between cerebral glutamate levels and the severity of symptoms in fibromyalgia patients[24]. Substance P is also markedly elevated in the cerebrospinal fluid of fibromyalgia patients[25]. Substance P is a neuropeptide that plays multiple major roles in the transmission of pain signals from the peripheral nervous system to the central nervous system. In contrast to a classical neurotransmitter like glutamate, substance P does not undergo rapid reuptake from the synaptic space but can travel farther locally and remain active for longer periods. Substance P mainly functions as a neuromodulator that sensitizes neurons and amplifies the actions of glutamate and thus boosts ascending pain signals[26]. Substance P has also been implicated in autonomic stress as well as the emotional stress response to pain[27].

Conversely, fibromyalgia patients have been shown to have decreased levels of γ-aminobutyric acid (GABA) in the anterior cingulate of the brain. GABA is the major inhibitory neurotransmitter of the central nervous system and plays a major role in pain processing[28]. Patients with fibromyalgia have also been shown to have reduced levels of monoaminergic neurotransmitters (serotonin, norepinephrine, and dopamine) in the cerebrospinal fluid[29].

Monoaminergic neurotransmitters play an important role in positive neuromodulation of the descending PAG-RVM pain control pathway thus, decreased monoamine levels can cause hyperalgesia through downregulation of descending central inhibition of pain signals [30,31]. Furthermore, reduced levels of these monoamines play an important role in the pathogenesis of psychiatric mood disorders. This relationship explains why depression is a common comorbidity that exacerbates the severity of chronic pain conditions like fibromyalgia[32].

Peripheral pain and fibromyalgia

Fibromyalgia is primarily regarded as a pathology of the central nervous system wherein mechanisms of localizing, processing, and inhibiting painful stimuli are dysregulated. However, the relationship between fibromyalgia and peripheral pain conditions has been studied and continues to be a field of interest. Fibromyalgia symptoms and disease activity are increased in patients with rheumatic peripheral pain conditions such as osteoarthritis, polymyositis, systemic lupus erythematosus, etc[33]. Furthermore, treatment of peripheral conditions can help with alleviating fibromyalgia symptoms[34]. This relationship remains to be understood from a pathophysiological perspective but is important to consider in clinical practice as accurately identifying and treating comorbid peripheral pain conditions is helpful in the management of patients with fibromyalgia.

From a peripheral nerve morphology perspective, patients with fibromyalgia have been shown to have reduced intradermal nerve diameter and density. However, there is no established correlation between pain and nerve density or diameter in these studies[35–37]. To our knowledge, there is no evidence to suggest whether these peripheral nerve changes are primary pathologies in fibromyalgia or whether they are adaptive mechanisms in response to the reduced descending inhibitory signals from the central nervous system. A study performed in mice showed that the administration of

Immunoglobulin G (IgG) from fibromyalgia patients in mice caused the mice to experience cold and pressure intolerance as well as reduced nerve fiber diameter. The IgG deposited in the dorsal root ganglia of the peripheral nervous system and administration of serum without IgG did not cause these symptoms in mice. This study indicates the possibility of autoimmune involvement in the peripheral nerve pathology observed in some fibromyalgia patients, but further studies are indicated to understand this relationship[38,39].

Conclusion

The pathophysiology of fibromyalgia is complicated and likely involves dysregulation of different brain signaling pathways, neurotransmitter levels, neuroreceptor activity levels, endocrine and autoimmune disruption, and other potential factors. This disruption leads to an overall increased activation of threat, pain, and pain memory processing and anticipation systems and a decreased activation of pain soothing and regulation systems and manifests as widespread pain and non-specific stress symptoms like sleep disruption, fatigue, and cognitive and emotional distress. The most recent distillation of fibromyalgia pathophysiology is the integrative "Fibromyalgia: Imbalance of Threat and Soothing Systems (FITSS)" model proposed by Pinto et al[40]. This complexity has made it difficult to understand the directionality of these disruptions and whether each specific pathophysiological finding plays a role in the pathogenesis of this disease or if it is the disease that is causing these disruptions.

References:

1. Mezhov, V., Guymer, E. & Littlejohn, G. Central sensitivity and fibromyalgia. *Internal Medicine Journal* 51, 1990–1998 (2021).

2. Kosek, E. *et al.* Do we need a third mechanistic descriptor for chronic pain states? *Pain* 157, 1382–1386 (2016).

3. Gracely, R. H., Petzke, F., Wolf, J. M. & Clauw, D. J. Functional magnetic resonance imaging evidence of augmented pain processing in fibromyalgia. *Arthritis & Rheumatism* 46, 1333–1343 (2002).

4. Fitzcharles, M.-A. *et al.* Nociplastic pain: towards an understanding of prevalent pain conditions. *The Lancet* 397, 2098–2110 (2021).

5. Dehghan, M. *et al.* Coordinate-based (ALE) meta-analysis of brain activation in patients with fibromyalgia. *Hum Brain Mapp* 37, 1749–1758 (2016).

6. Meulders, A., Jans, A. & Vlaeyen, J. W. S. Differences in pain-related fear acquisition and generalization: an experimental study comparing patients with fibromyalgia and healthy controls. *Pain* 156, 108–122 (2015).

7. Russo, A. *et al.* Advanced visual network and cerebellar hyperresponsiveness to trigeminal nociception in migraine with aura. *J Headache Pain* 20, 46 (2019).

8. Tesic, I., Pigoni, A., Moltrasio, C., Brambilla, P. & Delvecchio, G. How does feeling pain look like in depression: A review of functional neuroimaging studies. *Journal of Affective Disorders* 339, 400–411 (2023).

9. Pagliusi, M. & Gomes, F. V. The Role of The Rostral Ventromedial Medulla in Stress Responses. *Brain Sci* 13, 776 (2023).

10. Truini, A. *et al.* Abnormal resting state functional connectivity of the periaqueductal grey in patients with fibromyalgia. *Clin Exp Rheumatol* 34, S129-133 (2016).

11. Sandström, A. *et al.* Dysfunctional Activation of the Dorsolateral Prefrontal Cortex During Pain Anticipation Is Associated With Altered Subsequent Pain Experience in Fibromyalgia Patients. *The Journal of Pain* 24, 1731–1743 (2023).

12. Cagnie, B. *et al.* Central sensitization in fibromyalgia? A systematic review on structural and functional brain MRI. *Seminars in Arthritis and Rheumatism* 44, 68–75 (2014).

13. Kim, D. J. *et al.* Altered White Matter Integrity in the Corpus Callosum in Fibromyalgia Patients Identified by Tract-Based Spatial Statistical Analysis. *Arthritis & Rheumatology* 66, 3190–3199 (2014).

14. Lo, Y.-C., Li, T. J. T., Lin, T.-C., Chen, Y.-Y. & Kang, J.-H. Microstructural Evidence of Neuroinflammation for Psychological Symptoms and Pain in Patients With Fibromyalgia. *J Rheumatol* 49, 942–947 (2022).

15. Feinberg, T., Sambamoorthi, U., Lilly, C. & Innes, K. K. Potential Mediators between Fibromyalgia and C-Reactive protein: Results from a Large U.S. Community Survey. *BMC Musculoskelet Disord* 18, 294 (2017).

16. Üçeyler, N., Häuser, W. & Sommer, C. Systematic review with meta-analysis: cytokines in fibromyalgia syndrome. *BMC Musculoskelet Disord* 12, 245 (2011).

17. Bote, M. E., García, J. J., Hinchado, M. D. & Ortega, E. Inflammatory/Stress Feedback Dysregulation in Women with Fibromyalgia. *Neuroimmunomodulation* 19, 343–351 (2012).

18. Behm, F. G. *et al.* Unique immunologic patterns in fibromyalgia. *BMC Clin Pathol* 12, 25 (2012).

19. Harris, R. E. *et al.* Decreased central mu-opioid receptor availability in fibromyalgia. *J Neurosci* 27, 10000–10006 (2007).

20. Salemi, S. *et al.* Up-regulation of δ-opioid receptors and κ-opioid receptors in the skin of fibromyalgia patients. *Arthritis & Rheumatism* 56, 2464–2466 (2007).

21. Goldenberg, D. L., Clauw, D. J., Palmer, R. E. & Clair, A. G. Opioid Use in Fibromyalgia. *Mayo Clinic Proceedings* 91, 640–648 (2016).

22. Bleakman, D., Alt, A. & Nisenbaum, E. S. Glutamate receptors and pain. *Seminars in Cell & Developmental Biology* 17, 592–604 (2006).

23. Sarzi-Puttini, P., Giorgi, V., Marotto, D. & Atzeni, F. Fibromyalgia: an update on clinical characteristics, aetiopathogenesis and treatment. *Nat Rev Rheumatol* 16, 645–660 (2020).

24. Pyke, T. L., Osmotherly, P. G. & Baines, S. Measuring Glutamate Levels in the Brains of Fibromyalgia Patients and a Potential Role for Glutamate in the Pathophysiology of Fibromyalgia Symptoms: A Systematic Review. *The Clinical Journal of Pain* 33, 944–954 (2017).

25. Russell, I. J. *et al.* Elevated cerebrospinal fluid levels of substance p in patients with the fibromyalgia syndrome. *Arthritis & Rheumatism* 37, 1593–1601 (1994).

26. Zieglgänsberger, W. Substance P and pain chronicity. *Cell Tissue Res* 375, 227–241 (2019).

27. Ebner, K., Sartori, S. & Singewald, N. Tachykinin Receptors as Therapeutic Targets in Stress-Related Disorders. *CPD* 15, 1647–1674 (2009).

28. Foerster, B. R. et al. Reduced insular γ-aminobutyric acid in fibromyalgia. *Arthritis & Rheumatism* 64, 579–583 (2012).

29. Russell, I. J., Vaeroy, H., Javors, M. & Nyberg, F. Cerebrospinal fluid biogenic amine metabolites in fibromyalgia/fibrositis syndrome and rheumatoid arthritis. *Arthritis & Rheumatism* 35, 550–556 (1992).

30. Bardin, L. The complex role of serotonin and 5-HT receptors in chronic pain. *Behavioural Pharmacology* 22, 390–404 (2011).

31. Bannister, K. & Dickenson, A. H. What do monoamines do in pain modulation? *Curr Opin Support Palliat Care* 10, 143–148 (2016).

32. Bonilla-Jaime, H. et al. Depression and Pain: Use of Antidepressants. *Curr Neuropharmacol* 20, 384–402 (2022).

33. Haliloglu, S., Carlioglu, A., Akdeniz, D., Karaaslan, Y. & Kosar, A. Fibromyalgia in patients with other rheumatic diseases: prevalence and relationship with disease activity. *Rheumatol Int* 34, 1275–1280 (2014).

34. Affaitati, G. et al. Effects of treatment of peripheral pain generators in fibromyalgia patients. *European Journal of Pain* 15, 61–69 (2011).

35. Üçeyler, N. et al. Small fibre pathology in patients with fibromyalgia syndrome. *Brain* 136, 1857–1867 (2013).

36. Doppler, K., Rittner, H. L., Deckart, M. & Sommer, C. Reduced dermal nerve fiber diameter in skin biopsies of patients with fibromyalgia. *Pain* 156, 2319–2325 (2015).

37. Caro, X. J. & Winter, E. F. Evidence of Abnormal Epidermal Nerve Fiber Density in Fibromyalgia: Clinical and Immunologic Implications. *Arthritis & Rheumatology* 66, 1945–1954 (2014).

38. Martínez-Lavín, M. Dorsal root ganglia: fibromyalgia pain factory? *Clin Rheumatol* 40, 783–787 (2021).

39. Goebel, A. *et al.* Passive transfer of fibromyalgia symptoms from patients to mice. *Journal of Clinical Investigation* 131, e144201 (2021).

40. Pinto, A. M. *et al.* Neurophysiological and psychosocial mechanisms of fibromyalgia: A comprehensive review and call for an integrative model. *Neuroscience & Biobehavioral Reviews* 151, 105235 (2023).

Risk Factors of Fibromyalgia

George Yacoub

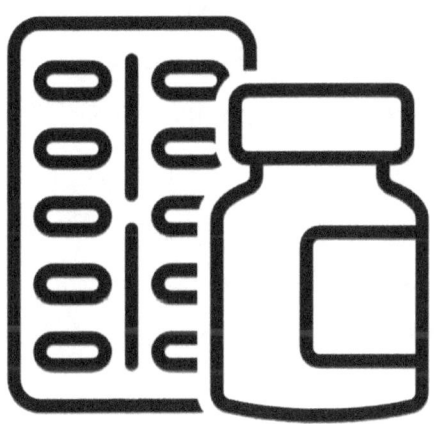

Biopsychosocial Model of Fibromyalgia

To encapsulate and comprehensively understand and manage the wide variety of risk factors and symptoms associated with fibromyalgia, clinicians are beginning to approach this disease using the biopsychosocial model. This model ascertains that to reach an adequate understanding of fibromyalgia, we must understand the higher-order psychosocial context in which patients perceive, process, and appraise biological stimuli that they interpret as pain. This is in addition to the understanding of the biological stimuli and pathways that are being interpreted and processed by the patient's mind. The complex pathophysiological findings observed in fibromyalgia support this approach as it indicates that this disease experience is likely a culmination of various factors rather than a specific pathophysiological phenomenon[1,2]. A meta-analysis by Creed et al. evaluating the non-genetic risk factors for fibromyalgia reports musculoskeletal disorders and other medical disorders like peptic ulcer disease, sleep disorders, diabetes, hypertension, and hyperlipidemia to all be associated with increased risk of fibromyalgia occurrence.

Furthermore, demographic and lifestyle factors like female sex, reduced number of years of formal education, stress, older and middle age, smoking, and raised BMI are associated with increased occurrence of fibromyalgia. A bidirectional relationship was found between fibromyalgia and depression, gastroesophageal reflux disorder, headache, migraine, insomnia, and irritable bowel syndrome (IBS)[3]. The role of psychiatric disorders in fibromyalgia is being increasingly recognized as another systematic review in 2021 conducted by

Kleykamp et al. found depression to be the most prevalent fibromyalgia comorbidity, with a lifetime prevalence of over 52%, followed by panic disorder, with a lifetime prevalence of 33%, bipolar disorder, with a lifetime prevalence of 26%, and PTSD, with a lifetime prevalence of 16% in fibromyalgia patients[4]. In addition to the effects of mood disorders on the risk of developing fibromyalgia, depression has been associated with increased pain hypersensitivity and cognitive fibromyalgia symptoms[5]. Some studies provide evidence to attribute the cognitive impairment associated with fibromyalgia to the depressive symptoms that commonly accompany fibromyalgia, as opposed to being a primary symptom of fibromyalgia[6]. Furthermore, fibromyalgia patients have a reduced capacity for regulating emotions; and emotional rejection, "an individual's tendency not to accept reactions that make them feel uncomfortable," and life interference, "difficulty in concentrating or performing tasks when experiencing negative emotional mood states," were shown to be independent predictors of pain severity in fibromyalgia patients[7]. A meta-analysis by Afari et al. suggests that adverse life events and trauma significantly increase the likelihood of developing fibromyalgia[8]. This study acknowledges its limitation in looking at retrospective and cross-sectional studies, which are all impacted by hindsight and recall bias, especially considering the topic of trauma recall. A prospective study by Kivimaki et al. assessing the impact of workplace stress on the risk of developing fibromyalgia also suggests that increased workplace stress is associated with an increased risk of developing fibromyalgia later on[9]. Negative affect and stress are proposed to alter pain sensitivity through many mechanisms, including HPA axis dysregulation, which some studies have explored in fibromyalgia with mixed results and conclusions, epigenetic modification of genes, inflammation, sleep, and circadian rhythm disruption, and disruption of descending pain inhibition pathways[2,10]. These results support a bidirectional model wherein patients with fibromyalgia experience pain hypersensitivity and upregulated negative affect and stress response mechanisms. The negative effect creates a cognitive ecosystem that has reduced the ability to appropriately inhibit, process, and modulate pain signals, which in turn upregulate the stress response[11]. In addition to amplification of pain stimuli and blunting descending inhibition of pain, upregulated negative affect is being recognized as a player in other fibromyalgia symptoms like sleep disorder and the cognitive symptoms of fibromyalgia[2]. Supporting this model are studies exploring and providing evidence for the effectiveness of positive affect in modulating pain and cognitive symptoms of chronic pain conditions[12,13]. Later sections will discuss the role of therapy and treatment of comorbid psychiatric conditions in the management of fibromyalgia.

Heritability and Associated Genetic Polymorphisms

As described in the previous chapter, the pathophysiology of fibromyalgia is not entirely understood, and there are no validated biomarkers or tests that can confidently confirm the diagnosis of fibromyalgia. This has made it difficult to pinpoint genetic traits or risk factors that make individuals more susceptible to this condition, and more research is needed in this field[14]. Familial linkage studies have shown that there is an 8-13 fold increase in risk of developing fibromyalgia if you have a first-degree relative with the condition[15,16].

This makes the possibility of finding genetic associations with this condition more promising. Several studies have focused on the role of *COMT (catechol-O-methyltransferase)* gene polymorphisms in fibromyalgia. COMT enzyme plays an important role in breaking down catecholamines, including dopamine, whose role in pain sensitization has been described in the previous section. A recent meta-analysis by Vetterlein et al. suggests that chronic pain patients homozygous for the COMT polymorphism *rs4680* experience increased pain sensitivity when compared to heterozygotes. It is important that this effect of *rs4680* on pain sensitivity was only observed when healthy patients (those not given a chronic pain diagnosis) were removed from the sample analysis. This indicates that this polymorphism might play a supportive role in amplifying the symptoms of fibromyalgia but is likely not sufficient to cause the pathology on its own. Combinations of different polymorphisms within the COMT gene were categorized into haplotype blocks labeled LPS for low pain sensitivity, APS for average pain sensitivity, and HPS for high pain sensitivity. These haplotype blocks were studied and found to have a significant effect on pain sensitivity in healthy patients[17]. These results were confirmed by the meta-analysis that shows pain sensitivity is significantly higher in patients homozygous for APS and LPS/HPS heterozygotes when compared to patients homozygous for LPS and APS/LPS heterozygotes. This effect was observed in the pooled patient sample that included patients with and without a chronic pain diagnosis[18]. These results indicate the importance of conducting more complex studies to evaluate the effects of different combinations of polymorphisms within different genes associated with pain and combinations of polymorphisms between different genetic loci rather than assessing the effects of individual gene polymorphisms[17,18].

Several studies have found associations between fibromyalgia and different genes involved in the regulation of serotonin as well. Specifically, mutations in *solute carrier family six member 4 (SCL6A4)*, involved in serotonin reuptake, *5-hydroxytryptamine receptor 2A (5-HTR2A)*, and *5-hydroxytryptamine receptor 3A (5-HTR3a)*, which are both serotonin receptors, have been associated with fibromyalgia and increased pain[19–23]. A cross-sectional study found an association between the *rs28358579* polymorphism in mitochondrial DNA and fibromyalgia. This polymorphism occurs in the 16S subunit of mitochondrial rRNA and in the 5'UTR of the human gene, which has anti-apoptotic and neuroprotective properties. This mutation, however, has not been sufficiently studied, and effects on human gene expression or rRNA structure are not established[24]. A cross-sectional study looking into the transient receptor potential vanilloid (TRPV) family of cation channels, known to play a role in afferent pain signaling, found no associations between specific *TRPV* gene polymorphisms and fibromyalgia susceptibility but a specific GTA haplotype of *TRPV2* was associated with decreased fibromyalgia susceptibility. Furthermore, this study showed an association between the rs395357 polymorphism of *TRPV3* and the severity of fibromyalgia symptoms[25]. A small cross-sectional study looking at the *Synaptosomal-associated protein of 25kDa (SNAP-25)* is a protein that is part of the SNARE complex and plays a role in synaptic vesicle fusion and neurotransmitter release. They found that the *rs1051312* polymorphism of the *SNAP-25* gene is associated with fibromyalgia diagnosis and increased depression and pain sensitivity symptoms[26]. *Guanosine triphosphate cyclohydrolase 1 (GCH1)* is an enzyme that plays a role in dopamine and serotonin biosynthesis, and a cross-sectional study found no significant association between specific polymorphisms in the *GCH1* gene and the occurrence of fibromyalgia or pain symptoms. However, haplotype analysis revealed that the CCTA haplotype for the following respective single nucleotide polymorphisms *rs841, rs752688, rs4411417, and rs3783641* was associated with lower pain sensitivity and frequency among fibromyalgia patients compared to the CCTT haplotype[27]. A much larger cross-sectional study by Smith et al. that included over 800 patients and looked at over 350 genes found an association between fibromyalgia and increased frequency of the *rs6454674* SNP in the *CB-1 cannabinoid receptor (CNR1)* gene and the *rs8192619* SNP in the *trace amine-associated receptor 1 (TAAR1)* gene. *TAAR1* is a g-protein coupled receptor that has been shown to play a role in dopamine uptake[28]. In a replication cohort using different genotyping assays, Smith et al. were able to confirm an association between fibromyalgia and flanking SNPs linked to the *rs8192619* SNP of *TAAR1*: *rs4129256* and *rs2745428*. They also confirmed an association between fibromyalgia and upstream promoter region SNPs that showed linkage to the *rs6454674* SNP of *CNR1*: *rs1078602* and *rs10485171*. While Smith et al. found strong associations between fibromyalgia and increased frequency of SNPs in other genes, these results were not consistently observed in their replication study[29]. These studies generally suffer from small sample sizes, and thus low power, and meta-analyses have failed to consistently confirm these associations. Therefore, there is currently no consensus on one particular gene mutation that has been universally accepted to accurately predict a significant increase in the risk of developing fibromyalgia[14]. The genetic component of fibromyalgia is complicated and likely involves gene-gene interactions of multiple genes that each occur in multiple genetic polymorphism haplotypes and haplotype blocks that result in the pathologic phenotype of fibromyalgia. There is an added layer of complexity due to epigenetic interactions that play an important role in fibromyalgia.

Epigenetics

In addition to genetic polymorphisms, there has been an increasing interest in understanding the epigenetic modifications associated with fibromyalgia and its symptoms[14,23]. Methylation of CpG islands in the promoter region of genes is one of the most well-understood epigenetic modifications that can reduce the expression of the downstream gene. Gerra et al. conducted a study looking at DNA methylation in over 100 different genomic methylation sites previously found associated with fibromyalgia, chronic widespread pain, depression, and other psychiatric disorders in fibromyalgia patients and healthy related sisters.

They found hypermethylation of the promoter region in the *GRM2* gene to be associated with fibromyalgia. *GRM2* codes for the type-2 metabotropic glutamate receptors (mGluR2), an inhibitory autoreceptor that modulates glutamatergic signaling throughout the central and peripheral nervous system. Hypermethylation of this gene is hypothesized to decrease expression of this inhibitory auto receptor and thus increase glutamate activity and indirectly reduce GABA and dopamine signaling. An epigenome-wide association study by Andrade et al. identified differentially methylated sites in patients diagnosed with fibromyalgia in the following genomic sites: 1p34, 6p21, 10q26, 17q25, and 19q13. Analysis of the CpG island-controlled genes in these sites revealed that fibromyalgia patients had significantly hypomethylated, and thus downregulated, genes involved in DNA repair pathways, immune system-related processes, metabolism related to lipids, and membrane transport. This indicates that these epigenetic modifications are likely a result of the upregulated cellular and autonomic system response to stress[30]. A similar analysis by Menzies et al. revealed genes with differentially methylated sites in fibromyalgia patients were associated with chromatin compaction, DNA damage/repair or chromosomal segregation, muscle contraction, axonal bundling, and outgrowth, cell signaling in muscle, neuronal excitability, muscle maturation, and response to oxidative stress[31]. Micro-RNA (miRNA) is a post-transcriptional method of repressing gene expression by inhibiting the translation of specific genes. Multiple studies have identified various micro-RNAs as being significantly associated with the development and symptoms of fibromyalgia (FM). A study by Hussein et al. found elevated levels of miRNA-320a in fibromyalgia patients and a positive correlation between miRNA-320a levels and symptom severity and duration. miRNA-320a has been implicated in regulating cellular metabolism, inflammation, and neuronal growth[32]. Other studies have found a negative correlation between fibromyalgia and several miRNAs implicated in cellular metabolism, neuronal development and growth, cell cycle control, and inflammation in fibromyalgia patients.

However, the direction of the relationship between epigenetic modification and fibromyalgia occurrence and symptoms requires further exploration as it is possible that one of the outcomes of the increased and dysregulated stress response seen in fibromyalgia patients results in the observed epigenetic modifications and resultant differential expression of genes[33,34].

Conclusion

Similarly to the pathogenesis of fibromyalgia, the risk factors associated with fibromyalgia are also challenging to parse out and understand as independent components. This is likely due to the complexity and heterogeneity of disease processes and symptoms that characterize fibromyalgia. There is certainly a heritable biological component that is involved in fibromyalgia, and that is demonstrated by the prevalence of the disease among people with first-degree relatives who have the disease. However, this genetic component is complicated by undeniable psychosocial contributions to the risk of developing fibromyalgia.

These psychosocial factors play a crucial role in amplifying the neuronal and emotional processing of biological stimuli and thus increasing the symptoms experienced by fibromyalgia patients, but they are also implicated in upregulating cellular and autonomic stress responses that result in epigenetic modification of target genes associated with fibromyalgia.

References:

1. Turk, D. C. & Adams, L. M. Using a Biopsychosocial Perspective in the Treatment of Fibromyalgia Patients. Pain Manag. 6, 357–369 (2016).
2. Pinto, A. M. et al. Neurophysiological and psychosocial mechanisms of fibromyalgia: A comprehensive review and call for an integrative model. Neuroscience & Biobehavioral Reviews 151, 105235 (2023).
3. Creed, F. A review of the incidence and risk factors for fibromyalgia and chronic widespread pain in population-based studies. Pain 161, 1169–1176 (2020).
4. Kleykamp, B. A. et al. The Prevalence of Psychiatric and Chronic Pain Comorbidities in Fibromyalgia: an ACTTION systematic review. Seminars in Arthritis and Rheumatism 51, 166–174 (2021).
5. Aguglia, A., Salvi, V., Maina, G., Rossetto, I. & Aguglia, E. Fibromyalgia syndrome and depressive symptoms: Comorbidity and clinical correlates. Journal of Affective Disorders 128, 262–266 (2011).
6. Gelonch, O. et al. The effect of depressive symptoms on cognition in patients with fibromyalgia. PLoS ONE 13, e0200057 (2018).
7. Trucharte, A. et al. Emotional regulation processes: influence on pain and disability in fibromyalgia patients. Clin Exp Rheumatol 38 Suppl 123, 40–46 (2020).
8. Afari, N. et al. Psychological Trauma and Functional Somatic Syndromes: A Systematic Review and Meta-Analysis. Psychosomatic Medicine 76, 2–11 (2014).

9. Kivimaki, M. et al. Work stress and incidence of newly diagnosed fibromyalgia. Journal of Psychosomatic Research 57, 417–422 (2004).

10. Agorastos, A., Pervanidou, P., Chrousos, G. P. & Baker, D. G. Developmental Trajectories of Early Life Stress and Trauma: A Narrative Review on Neurobiological Aspects Beyond Stress System Dysregulation. Front. Psychiatry 10, 118 (2019).

11. Peters, M. L. Emotional and Cognitive Influences on Pain Experience. in Modern Trends in Psychiatry (eds. Finn, D. P. & Leonard, B. E.) vol. 30 138–152 (S. Karger AG, 2015).

12. Finan, P. H. & Garland, E. L. The Role of Positive Affect in Pain and Its Treatment. The Clinical Journal of Pain 31, 177–187 (2015).

13. Hanssen, M. M., Peters, M. L., Boselie, J. J. & Meulders, A. Can positive affect attenuate (persistent) pain? State of the art and clinical implications. Curr Rheumatol Rep 19, 80 (2017).

14. D'Agnelli, S. et al. Fibromyalgia: Genetics and epigenetics insights may provide the basis for the development of diagnostic biomarkers. Mol Pain 15, 1744806918819944 (2019).

15. Arnold, L. M. et al. Family study of fibromyalgia. Arthritis & Rheumatism 50, 944–952 (2004).

16. Arnold, L. M. et al. The Fibromyalgia Family Study: A Genome-Wide Linkage Scan Study. Arthritis & Rheumatism 65, 1122–1128 (2013).

17. Diatchenko, L. et al. Catechol- O -methyltransferase gene polymorphisms are associated with multiple pain-evoking stimuli. Pain 125, 216–224 (2006).

18. Vetterlein, A., Monzel, M. & Reuter, M. Are catechol-O-methyltransferase gene polymorphisms genetic markers for pain sensitivity after all? – A review and meta-analysis. Neuroscience & Biobehavioral Reviews 148, 105112 (2023).

19. Estévez-López, F. et al. Interplay between genetics and lifestyle on pain susceptibility in women with fibromyalgia: the al-Ándalus project. Rheumatology 61, 3180–3191 (2022).

20. Ledermann, K. et al. 5′UTR polymorphism in the serotonergic receptor HTR3A gene is differently associated with striatal Dopamine D2/D3 receptor availability in the right putamen in Fibromyalgia patients and healthy controls—Preliminary evidence. Synapse 74, e22147 (2020).

21. Vargas-Alarcón, G. et al. Association of adrenergic receptor gene polymorphisms with different fibromyalgia syndrome domains. Arthritis & Rheumatism 60, 2169–2173 (2009).

22. Lee, Y. H., Choi, S. J., Ji, J. D. & Song, G. G. Candidate gene studies of fibromyalgia: a systematic review and meta-analysis. Rheumatol Int 32, 417–426 (2012).

23. Ovrom, E. A. et al. A Comprehensive Review of the Genetic and Epigenetic Contributions to the Development of Fibromyalgia. Biomedicines 11, 1119 (2023).

24. van Tilburg, M. A. L. et al. A genetic polymorphism that is associated with mitochondrial energy metabolism increases risk of fibromyalgia. Pain 161, 2860–2871 (2020).

25. Park, D.-J. et al. Polymorphisms of the TRPV2 and TRPV3 genes associated with fibromyalgia in a Korean population. Rheumatology 55, 1518–1527 (2016).

26. Balkarli, A., Sengül, C., Tepeli, E., Balkarli, H. & Cobankara, V. Synaptosomal-associated protein 25 (Snap-25) gene polymorphism frequency in fibromyalgia syndrome and relationship with clinical symptoms. BMC Musculoskelet Disord 15, 191 (2014).

27. Kim, S.-K. et al. Association of Guanosine Triphosphate Cyclohydrolase 1 Gene Polymorphisms with Fibromyalgia Syndrome in a Korean Population. J Rheumatol 40, 316–322 (2013).

28. Miller, G. M. The emerging role of trace amine-associated receptor 1 in the functional regulation of monoamine transporters and dopaminergic activity. J Neurochem 116, 164–176 (2011).

29. Smith, S. B. et al. Large candidate gene association study reveals genetic risk factors and therapeutic targets for fibromyalgia. Arthritis Rheum 64, 584–593 (2012).

30. Ciampi De Andrade, D. et al. Epigenetics insights into chronic pain: DNA hypomethylation in fibromyalgia—a controlled pilot-study. Pain 158, 1473–1480 (2017).

31. Menzies, V. et al. Epigenetic alterations and an increased frequency of micronuclei in women with fibromyalgia. Nurs Res Pract 2013, 795784 (2013).

32. Hussein, M. et al. The Impact of Micro RNA-320a Serum Level on Severity of Symptoms and Cerebral Processing of Pain in Patients with Fibromyalgia. Pain Medicine 23, 2061–2072 (2022).

33. Cerdá-Olmedo, G., Mena-Durán, A. V., Monsalve, V. & Oltra, E. Identification of a MicroRNA Signature for the Diagnosis of Fibromyalgia. PLoS ONE 10, e0121903 (2015).

34. Bjersing, J. L., Lundborg, C., Bokarewa, M. I. & Mannerkorpi, K. Profile of Cerebrospinal microRNAs in Fibromyalgia. PLoS ONE 8, e78762 (2013).

Non-pharmacological management of fibromyalgia

Natalie Soliman

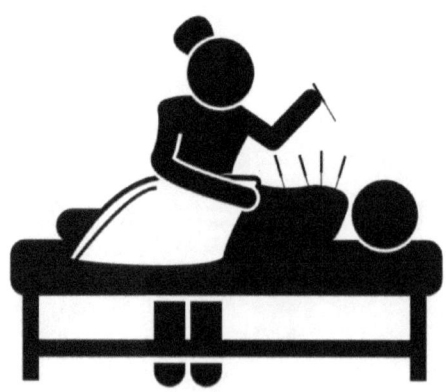

Introduction:

Fibromyalgia (FM) is a syndrome characterized by chronic musculoskeletal pain that can be felt in different parts of the body.[1] To put it simply, it is a condition marked by ongoing muscle and joint pain that can affect various parts of the body. The main symptoms of the disease are widespread musculoskeletal pain, muscle and joint stiffness, insomnia, fatigue, mood disorders, cognitive dysfunction, anxiety, depression, general sensitivity, and inability to perform daily activities[2-3].

Effective management often involves a combination of pharmacological and non-pharmacological approaches. Many international health organizations advocate for the inclusion of drug-free treatments alongside medications and sometimes even recommend these as the first line of treatment.

In 2017, the European Alliance of Associations for Rheumatology (EULAR) updated its recommendations for managing fibromyalgia based on scientific evidence from high-quality reviews and meta-analyses[4]. As a first-line approach, EULAR recommended educating patients and starting with non-pharmacological therapies such as aerobic and strengthening exercises. These can be combined with other non-drug therapies like cognitive behavioral therapy, acupuncture, hydrotherapy, massage, meditative movement therapies, and mindfulness-based stress reduction.

This chapter will explore various non-pharmacological treatment options, drawing on literature reviews and evidence-based reports.

Physical Therapy:

While medication mainly focuses on pain reduction, physical therapy is aimed at disease consequences such as pain, fatigue, deconditioning, muscle weakness, sleep disturbances, and other disease consequences[5]. In other words, medication targets the symptoms of pain directly, while physical therapy focuses on addressing the broader effects caused by fibromyalgia. Furthermore, no pharmacological intervention is effective in managing all FM symptoms, as they can only alleviate individual symptoms[6].

Physical exercise, the most strongly indicated nonpharmacological therapy, is based on aerobic exercises, resistance exercises for muscle strengthening, and stretching exercises[7]. Physical therapy, encompassing both passive and active techniques, can help prevent or reverse central sensitization, which is thought to contribute to chronic pain. Physical therapy and strengthening exercises work through several mechanisms, such as enhancing descending inhibition, correcting somatic dysfunctions, and optimizing sensory input patterns.

Their effects may involve modulating neural hypersensitivity, inflammation, and muscle dysfunction[9].

In essence, physical therapy improves the brain's ability to suppress pain signals, corrects musculoskeletal issues, and optimizes sensory input. Its benefits may include decreased nerve sensitivity, reduced inflammation, and enhanced muscle function.

Aerobic Exercise;

The American College of Sports Medicine (ACSM) defines aerobic exercise as any activity that uses large muscle groups, can be maintained continuously, and is rhythmic in nature[10]. This type of exercise relies on aerobic metabolism to produce energy (ATP) from amino acids, carbohydrates, and fatty acids. Examples of aerobic exercise include walking, hiking, cycling, dancing, jogging, long-distance running, and swimming. During aerobic exercise, the hypothalamus releases neurotransmitters, including endorphins, which help reduce pain. Increased levels of these neurotransmitters are also associated with better mood and improved sleep quality.

Numerous studies have demonstrated these benefits in practice. A 2022 systematic review of 18 studies concluded that aerobic exercise, resistance training, and stretching exercise have positive effects on pain, depression, and quality of life in adults with FM[11]. Another systematic review in 2023 analyzed 14 randomized controlled trials, with nine included in the final analysis[12]. The findings indicate that aerobic exercise is effective for pain management in fibromyalgia patients, proving more effective than stretching exercises. However, its effectiveness was similar to that of Pilates, muscle strengthening exercises, relaxation techniques, and stress management treatments.

Engaging in aerobic exercise for 30 to 60 minutes, 2 or 3 times a week, at an intensity of 50–80% of maximum heart rate, along with muscle-strengthening exercises (1 to 3 sets of 8–11 exercises, 8–10 repetitions per set, using a moderate weight), has been found to effectively reduce pain and severity in fibromyalgia patients when practiced consistently over 4 to 6 months[13]. Although there is no absolute consensus, it seems that 2 or 3 sessions of mild to moderate intensity physical activity, lasting 30–45 minutes each, are effective[13].

Tai Chi:

Tai Chi is an ancient Chinese practice that combines physical exercise with mind-body meditation, rooted in centuries-old traditions. It consists of slow, gentle movements and specific physical postures, fostering a meditative mindset and controlled breathing. This distinctive form of exercise involves movements primarily performed in a semi-squatting position. These movements require a continuous shift in the body's center of gravity, incorporating posture control, trunk rotation, weight transfer, and strength training[14-16]. All these features are advantageous for improving balance and strength, reducing the risk of falling, and the fear of falling[14-16].

A significant study by Wang et al. (2018) explored the effectiveness of Tai Chi compared to aerobic exercise in managing fibromyalgia symptoms[17]. The randomized, controlled trial included 226 adults with fibromyalgia and evaluated the impact of Tai Chi on various health outcomes over 52 weeks. Participants were assigned to either supervised aerobic exercise or one of four Tai Chi interventions varying in duration and frequency. The study found that Tai Chi was as effective, if not more so, than aerobic exercise in improving fibromyalgia symptoms. Key improvements were noted in the fibromyalgia impact questionnaire (FIQR) scores, patient's global assessment, anxiety levels, self-efficacy, and coping strategies. Notably, a longer duration of Tai Chi (24 weeks) resulted in greater benefits compared to a shorter duration (12 weeks). Additionally, participants demonstrated higher adherence to Tai Chi sessions than to aerobic exercise. These findings suggest that Tai Chi, with its low-impact and meditative approach, is a valuable therapeutic option for fibromyalgia patients, offering significant improvements in both physical and psychological symptoms.

Another recent study in 2024 aimed to evaluate the effectiveness of Traditional Chinese Exercise in reducing pain, improving sleep quality, and alleviating symptoms of anxiety and depression among fibromyalgia patients[18]. A systematic review of 15 randomized controlled trials involving 936 participants concluded that Traditional Chinese Exercise showed significant benefits compared to control interventions in these areas. The findings underscore the potential of Traditional Chinese Exercise as an effective treatment option for managing symptoms of fibromyalgia.

Overall, Tai Chi's traditional roots and gentle movements make it an appealing and accessible exercise for individuals with fibromyalgia, contributing to its potential as part of a multidisciplinary treatment plan.

Aquatic Therapy:

Aquatic therapy creates a fun therapy environment that utilizes water properties, such as natural resistance and buoyancy, to help patients improve their functionality. Immersion in warm water increases blood flow and, therefore, oxygen in the blood, eliminating catabolites and reducing the level of IL-8 and noradrenaline, which are responsible for activating nociceptors[19]. This means that being submerged in warm water increases blood circulation, leading to higher oxygen levels in the blood. This process helps remove harmful metabolic byproducts (catabolites) and reduces levels of substances like IL-8 and noradrenaline, which activate pain receptors (nociceptors). Thus, immersion in warm water can help alleviate pain and improve overall comfort. Additionally, warm water immersion reduces the activity of the sympathetic nervous system, potentially decreasing inflammation and pain perception in individuals with musculoskeletal disorders[20].

The benefits of aquatic therapy also stem from hydrostatic pressure, which reduces stress on the joints and enables functional exercises with less gravitational impact. This property allows for more intense exercise, strength, and range of motion with less cardiovascular stress[21].

The effectiveness of aquatic therapy has been assessed in a previous review published in 2013, showing beneficial effects on physical fitness, wellness, and symptoms associated with FM[22]. A study by Choy et al. indicated that sleep dysfunction may induce fibromyalgia-like symptoms and may have bidirectional roles in the pathophysiology of fibromyalgia[23]. Sleep quality is defined as an individual's self-satisfaction with all aspects of the sleep experience that can be measured by the following variables: sleep efficiency, sleep latency, wake after sleep onset, and sleep architecture measures[24]. This means that sleep quality refers to how satisfied someone is with their overall sleep experience. It's measured by factors like how efficiently they sleep, how long it takes to fall asleep, how often they wake up during the night and the pattern of their sleep stages.

In a 2023 systematic review and meta-analysis, researchers assessed the effectiveness of aquatic therapy for people with fibromyalgia by reviewing 22 randomized controlled trials from various databases up to October 2022[20]. The analysis found that aquatic therapy shows potential benefits for improving sleep quality and reducing pain in the short term, as measured by tools such as the Pittsburgh Sleep Quality Index and the Fibromyalgia Impact Questionnaire.

All in all, aquatic therapy appears to be effective as an additional treatment alongside standard care for managing symptoms of fibromyalgia, including pain and sleep quality.

Occupational Therapy:

Occupational therapy is a healthcare profession that focuses on helping people of all ages do the activities they want and need to do through therapeutic interventions. It aims to improve and maintain physical, cognitive, and emotional well-being by addressing barriers that may limit participation in daily life activities, such as self-care, work, leisure, and social interactions. Occupational therapists work with individuals to enhance their abilities, adapt to environments, and provide guidance on using specialized tools or techniques to achieve greater independence and quality of life.

A systematic review investigated the effectiveness of occupational therapy interventions for adults with fibromyalgia[25]. This review assessed studies published from January 2000 to June 2014, analyzing 322 abstracts from five databases. The interventions evaluated included cognitive-behavioral therapy, relaxation techniques, emotional disclosure, physical activity, and multidisciplinary approaches. These interventions showed strong evidence for improving daily activities, reducing pain, and alleviating depressive symptoms and fatigue.

A case report highlights how occupational therapy improved a patient with fibromyalgia[26]. It focuses on Jennifer, a 37-year-old teacher recently diagnosed with fibromyalgia, and how occupational therapy interventions were applied in her home setting. These interventions included developing a structured schedule for household tasks, using aquatic exercises for pain management and strength, mindfulness training for pain and depression, and connecting Jennifer with online and community support groups. By the end of 14 therapy sessions, Jennifer showed improvements in her ability to work and engage in leisure activities, with reduced symptoms of pain and depression.

Transcutaneous Electrical Nerve Stimulation (TENS):
Transcutaneous electrical nerve stimulation (TENS) is a non-invasive peripheral stimulation technique used to relieve pain by delivering pulsed electrical currents across the intact skin surface to activate underlying nerves. Patients can self-administer TENS and adjust the dosage as needed because there is no risk of overdose and few side effects or drug interactions. Maximal pain relief occurs when TENS produces a strong but non-painful electrical sensation (paresthesia) beneath the electrodes[27]. This means that TENS is a method to ease pain without surgery or inserting anything into the body.

TENS works by using a device to send mild electrical impulses through the skin to stimulate nerves underneath. These electrical impulses can modify or block pain signals sent to the brain, which may help reduce pain and promote healing in some cases. It is commonly used to treat various types of pain, including musculoskeletal pain, neuropathic pain, and certain types of chronic pain conditions. The effectiveness of TENS therapy also depends on where the electrodes are positioned. It is recommended to place the electrodes on healthy, sensitive skin so that the tingling sensation from TENS spreads across the painful area. This is typically done by directly placing the electrodes on or around the painful spot, known as 'bracketing' the area.

Contraindications include people who have cardiac pacemakers and implantable cardioverter defibrillators. Precautions include pregnancy, epilepsy, active malignancy, deep-vein thrombosis, and frail or damaged skin[28].

TENS has been evaluated in several studies as a non-pharmacological treatment for fibromyalgia. A review analyzed seven randomized controlled trials (RCTs) and one quasi-RCT involving 315 adults, primarily women[29]. While some of these studies indicated that TENS may effectively alleviate fibromyalgia pain, the reliability of these findings is limited by small sample sizes and diverse outcomes, which hindered the ability to combine results statistically. However, a study did find that a single 30-minute TENS treatment reduced movement-related pain and fatigue without serious adverse events reported[30]

Acupuncture:

Acupuncture therapy is an ancient practice rooted in traditional Chinese medicine, involving the insertion of fine needles into specific points on the body, known as acupuncture points. These points are believed to correspond to pathways called meridians, through which energy or "qi" flows. This therapeutic approach, with a history spanning over 2500 years, is based on the concept that disruptions in the flow of qi can contribute to illness. By stimulating these points, acupuncture aims to restore balance to the flow of energy and potentially bring about positive changes in physical, emotional, mental, and spiritual health. Ancient traditional Chinese medicine texts recognize a condition called the *Bi syndrome*, in which acupuncture is highly effective. This syndrome is similar to FM and consists of myofascial pain, arthralgia, and fatigue with varying manifestations[31].

The National Institute of Health Consensus Conference on Acupuncture concluded that acupuncture may be useful as an adjunct or alternative treatment for FM, or it may be included in a comprehensive management program for patients with FM[32]. Several randomized, controlled, and cohort studies have been published that show the beneficial effect of acupuncture for patients with FM[33-35]. In research conducted by Sprott et al., they studied 20 patients diagnosed with fibromyalgia (FM) who received acupuncture treatments tailored to their needs[34]. The study used laser flowmetry to examine blood flow at the five most significant tender points on the patients' bodies, comparing these results with temperature measurements and dolorimetry, a technique that assesses pain sensitivity. The findings indicated that acupuncture led to increased blood flow around all treated tender points, and the average number of sensitive points decreased from 16.1 to 13.8 following the acupuncture sessions. These results suggest that acupuncture may enhance blood circulation and reduce the number of painful tender points experienced by patients with fibromyalgia. Despite the positive results found, the number of publications related to the application of acupuncture is still scant, especially concerning FM treatment[31].

Laser Therapy:

The laser uses light energy; light consisting of coherent beams of single wavelengths has the potential to modulate cell/tissue physiology and to provide analgesic and/or anti-inflammatory effects in humans[36]. Photon energy from a laser also has the potential to oxidize the cytochrome c oxidase enzyme and then induce cellular oxygen metabolism. Increased muscle blood flow and oxygenation can assist in treating painful conditions[37]. This means that photon energy emitted by a laser can interact with certain enzymes in our cells, such as cytochrome c oxidase. This interaction can trigger a process that enhances how cells use oxygen for their energy needs. Consequently, there is an increase in blood flow to muscles and improved delivery of oxygen to these tissues. This enhanced oxygen supply can help alleviate pain associated with various conditions by supporting muscle function and reducing discomfort. Thus, laser therapy aims to enhance the body's natural healing processes through these mechanisms.

In a randomized, single-blind, placebo-controlled study, researchers assessed the effectiveness of 904 nm Gallium Arsenide low-energy laser therapy in 40 patients with fibromyalgia (FM)[38]. Patients were divided into active laser and placebo groups and treated daily for two weeks, excluding weekends. Both groups were evaluated for improvements in pain, number of tender points, skinfold tenderness, stiffness, sleep disturbance, fatigue, and muscular spasms. Significant improvements were observed in all parameters except sleep disturbance, fatigue, and skinfold tenderness in the placebo group. Before therapy, there were no significant differences between the two groups across all parameters. However, after therapy, the active laser group, which used a 904 nm Gallium Arsenide low-energy laser, showed significant improvements in pain, muscle spasm, morning stiffness, and total tender point numbers compared to the placebo group.

Based on these findings, the authors conclude that 904 nm Gallium Arsenide low energy laser therapy, a type of laser known for its specific wavelength and material composition, is effective in alleviating pain, muscle spasm, morning stiffness, and overall tender point count in patients with fibromyalgia. They suggest that this therapy is a safe and effective treatment option for individuals with fibromyalgia.

Electromagnetic Therapy:

Electromagnetic therapy involves using electromagnetic fields or waves to treat medical conditions. In a trial exploring a drug-free solution, participants used a wristband emitting millimeter waves alongside therapeutic coaching [39]. These waves were believed to modulate neural activity by stimulating endorphin release and activating the parasympathetic nervous system, potentially improving sleep quality, reducing anxiety, and alleviating pain. The study, conducted across eight French centers with 170 participants, evaluated the solution's effectiveness using the Fibromyalgia Impact Questionnaire over three months. Participants were randomly assigned to either an Immediate or

Delayed group to minimize bias. The Immediate group received the wristband alongside standard care immediately, while the Delayed group waited three months before receiving it, continuing with standard care in the interim. Real-time monitoring via a smartphone application tracked wristband usage, enhancing patient compliance. Though not double-blind due to the nature of the intervention, patient self-reports served as primary and secondary endpoints, ensuring data integrity. This innovative approach aimed to validate a non-medicinal treatment option that could significantly enhance the quality of life for fibromyalgia patients, aligning with recommendations for drug-free approaches in chronic pain management.

In another pilot study, researchers tested the effectiveness of extremely low-frequency magnetic field (ELF-MF) therapy in reducing chronic pain in fibromyalgia patients[40]. Thirty-seven women participated and were divided into two groups. Each group received both ELF-MF therapy and a sham treatment in different sequences. Pain and symptoms were measured at several points during the study. The results showed that ELF-MF therapy significantly reduced pain, although pain levels increased after stopping the therapy, they remained lower than before the treatment. The study suggests that ELF-MF therapy could be a helpful part of a broader treatment plan for managing fibromyalgia pain and improving the effectiveness of other treatments.

Cognitive Behavioral Therapy (CBT):
Cognitive Behavioral Therapy (CBT) is a short-term, goal-oriented psychotherapy focusing on changing thought patterns and behaviors, differing from classical psychoanalysis, which seeks deep insights.

Unlike the lengthy process of psychoanalysis, CBT can achieve beneficial effects within 10-20 sessions and can be conducted individually or in groups. Initially applied to mood disorders, CBT has expanded to address various medical conditions, including chronic pain states. Over the past 18 years, CBT has been used in several chronic pain treatment programs for fibromyalgia[41].

A study investigated the impact of Internet-based cognitive-behavioral therapy (ICBT) on women diagnosed with fibromyalgia[42]. Sixty participants were randomly assigned to three groups: traditional cognitive-behavioral therapy (CBT), ICBT, and a control group. Each intervention group consisted of 20 individuals. The CBT and ICBT groups attended ten weekly sessions lasting 2 hours each. The content of both types of sessions included progressive muscle relaxation, breathing techniques, problem-solving strategies, cognitive restructuring, psychoeducation about fibromyalgia and its symptoms, pain management techniques, and addressing sexual dysfunction issues. In the CBT group, sessions were conducted by a PhD in Clinical Psychology and a Master of Psychology, while in the ICBT group, sessions were led by a psychiatrist and a Master of Psychology through online platforms. The control group initially did not receive any specific intervention but was offered CBT sessions two months after the conclusion of the study's intervention period. After treatment, only the CBT group showed improvement in the primary outcome measure. Both the CBT and iCBT groups demonstrated reductions in psychological distress, depression, catastrophizing, and increased use of relaxation as a coping strategy. The ICBT group specifically showed improvements in self-efficacy, which were not observed in the CBT group. At follow-up, ICBT was more effective than CBT alone. Members of the ICBT group continued to show improvements in their scores at 6- and 12-month follow-ups. By the 12-month follow-up, the iCBT group surpassed their initial scores on the primary outcome measure and catastrophizing levels observed post-treatment. While CBT was expected to have similar effects, the positive results seen immediately after treatment were not sustained at follow-up.

These findings suggest that ICBT may enhance certain factors, such as self-efficacy and catastrophizing, compared to traditional CBT. The interactive nature of ICBT potentially facilitates social support, which could improve treatment adherence over time. Additionally, Turk et al. suggested that CBT might be most successful in a subgroup of fibromyalgia patients with prominent psychological distress and dysfunctional patterns of thinking and behavior[43].

In conclusion, the current evidence provides modest support for the use of CBT in the management of fibromyalgia, especially when it is part of a more comprehensive program utilizing medications and exercise[44].

Mindfulness:

Mindfulness meditation, originating from ancient Buddhist philosophy, has transformed into psychological and medical practices aimed at providing short-term therapeutic benefits[45]. Mindfulness-based stress reduction (MBSR) and mindfulness-based cognitive therapy (MBCT), derived from Buddhist traditions, are widely used to manage chronic pain and depression, respectively. These approaches have demonstrated effectiveness in improving mental health, reducing stress, and alleviating somatic symptoms.

Nonpharmacological interventions, such as mindfulness, are safer and more acceptable than medications for persons with fibromyalgia[46]. A study investigated the effectiveness of Mindfulness-Based Cognitive Therapy (MBCT) in alleviating the impact of fibromyalgia, depressive symptoms, and pain intensity among women with fibromyalgia[47]. Conducted with a pre-post treatment design and a 3-month follow-up, 33 female patients were randomly assigned to either the MBCT group or a control condition. The 8-week MBCT intervention aimed to reduce fibromyalgia impact, depressive symptoms (measured using the Fibromyalgia Impact Questionnaire and Beck Depression Inventory), and pain intensity (measured via Visual Analogue Scale). Results indicated significant reductions in the impact of fibromyalgia and depressive symptoms immediately after treatment, with these improvements maintained at the 3-month follow-up. The findings suggest that MBCT may effectively reduce depressive symptoms and improve the overall impact of fibromyalgia in affected women.

In another on fibromyalgia patients, researchers tested an 8-week mindfulness program called mindfulness-based stress reduction (MBSR)[48]. They divided 177 women into three groups: one receiving MBSR, another an active control, and a third on a waitlist. The main focus was on health-related quality of life (HRQoL) after 2 months. The results showed no big differences between the groups initially, but overall, HRQoL improved slightly (P=0.004). Only the MBSR group saw significant improvements in HRQoL (P=0.02) after the program. Secondary measures also showed some benefits for MBSR, including improvements in 6 out of 8 areas studied, compared to 3 for the active control and 2 for the waitlist.

Furthermore, a study aimed to explore the effects of a breathing exercises program on pain thresholds at tender points and daily life impact in women with fibromyalgia (FM)[49]. Thirty-five participants were randomly assigned to either an exercise group, performing 30-minute sessions daily for 12 weeks, or a control group. Pain thresholds and FM impact were assessed using an algometer and the Fibromyalgia Impact Questionnaire (FIQ). After 12 weeks, the exercise group showed significant improvements in pain thresholds, functional capacity, pain, and fatigue compared to the control group. Specific tender points like the second rib, occiput, and supraspinatus predicted these improvements. The findings suggest that breathing exercises are an effective intervention for managing FM symptoms in women.

Nutrition:

Several articles highlight the advantages of providing appropriate nutritional guidance to individuals with fibromyalgia (FM). Thus, after following a diet rich in antioxidant nutrients, clinical improvement in FM symptoms was reported[50]. Recent studies suggest that deficiencies in essential nutrients like amino acids, magnesium, selenium, and vitamins B and D may contribute to FM symptoms, including impaired pain regulation mechanisms[51]. Furthermore, heavy metals such as mercury, cadmium, and lead have also been linked to FM, potentially affecting nutrient absorption and exacerbating symptoms. Addressing nutritional imbalances through dietary adjustments is crucial for FM patients, as achieving optimal nutrient levels has been shown to reduce pain levels.

References:

1. Siracusa R, Paola RD, Cuzzocrea S, Impellizzeri D. Fibromyalgia: Pathogenesis, Mechanisms, Diagnosis and Treatment Options Update. Int J Mol Sci. 2021 Apr 9;22(8):3891. doi: 10.3390/ijms22083891. PMID: 33918736; PMCID: PMC8068842.

2. Gerdle B, Björk J, Cöster L, Henriksson K, Henriksson C, Bengtsson A. Prevalence of widespread pain and associations with work status: a population study. BMC Musculoskelet Disord. 2008 Jul 15; 9:102. Doi: 10.1186/1471-2474-9-102. PMID: 18627605; PMCID: PMC2488345.

3. Bennett RM, Jones J, Turk DC, Russell IJ, Matallana L. An internet survey of 2,596 people with fibromyalgia. BMC Musculoskelet Disord. 2007 Mar 9; 8:27. Doi: 10.1186/1471-2474-8-27. PMID: 17349056; PMCID: PMC1829161.

4. Macfarlane GJ, Kronisch C, Dean LE, Atzeni F, Häuser W, Fluß E, Choy E, Kosek E, Amris K, Branco J, Dincer F, Leino-Arjas P, Longley K, McCarthy GM, Makri S, Perrot S, Sarzi-Puttini P, Taylor A, Jones GT. EULAR revised recommendations for the management of fibromyalgia. Ann Rheum Dis. 2017 Feb;76(2):318-328. doi: 10.1136/annrheumdis-2016-209724. Epub 2016 Jul 4. PMID: 27377815

5. Offenbächer M, Stucki G. Physical therapy in the treatment of fibromyalgia. Scand J Rheumatol Suppl. 2000; 113:78-85. doi: 10.1080/030097400446706. PMID: 11028838.

6. Chen J, Han B, Wu C. On the superiority of a combination of aerobic and resistance exercise for fibromyalgia syndrome: A network meta-analysis. Front Psychol. 2022 Sep 28; 13:949256. Doi: 10.3389/fpsyg.2022.949256. PMID: 36248603; PMCID: PMC9554347.

7. Macfarlane GJ, Kronisch C, Dean LE, Atzeni F, Häuser W, Fluß E, Choy E, Kosek E, Amris K, Branco J, Dincer F, Leino-Arjas P, Longley K, McCarthy GM, Makri S, Perrot S, Sarzi-Puttini P, Taylor A, Jones GT. EULAR revised recommendations for the management of fibromyalgia. Ann Rheum Dis. 2017 Feb;76(2):318-328. doi: 10.1136/annrheumdis-2016-209724. Epub 2016 Jul 4. PMID: 27377815.

8. Van Griensven H, Schmid A, Trendafilova T, Low M. Central Sensitization in Musculoskeletal Pain: Lost in Translation? J Orthop Sports Phys Ther. 2020 Nov;50(11):592-596. doi: 10.2519/jospt.2020.0610. PMID: 33131390.

9. Schulze NB, Salemi MM, de Alencar GG, Moreira MC, de Siqueira GR. Efficacy of Manual Therapy on Pain, Impact of Disease, and Quality of Life in the Treatment of Fibromyalgia: A Systematic Review. Pain Physician. 2020 Sep;23(5):461-476. PMID: 32967389.

10. Wahid A, Manek N, Nichols M, Kelly P, Foster C, Webster P, Kaur A, Friedemann Smith C, Wilkins E, Rayner M, Roberts N, Scarborough P. Quantifying the Association Between Physical Activity and Cardiovascular Disease and Diabetes: A Systematic Review and Meta-Analysis. J Am Heart Assoc. 2016 Sep 14;5(9):e002495. doi: 10.1161/JAHA.115.002495. PMID:

27628572; PMCID: PMC5079002.

11. Couto N, Monteiro D, Cid L, Bento T. Effect of different types of exercise in adult subjects with fibromyalgia: a systematic review and meta-analysis of randomized clinical trials. Sci Rep. 2022 Jun 20;12(1):10391. doi: 10.1038/s41598-022-14213-x. PMID: 35725780; PMCID: PMC9209512.

12. Manojlović D, Kopše EI. The effectiveness of aerobic exercise for pain management in patients with fibromyalgia. Eur J Transl Myol. 2023 Jul 14;33(3):11423. doi: 10.4081/ejtm.2023.11423. PMID: 37449965; PMCID: PMC10583145.

13. Sosa-Reina MD, Nunez-Nagy S, Gallego-Izquierdo T, Pecos-Martín D, Monserrat J, Álvarez-Mon M. Effectiveness of Therapeutic Exercise in Fibromyalgia Syndrome: A Systematic Review and Meta-Analysis of Randomized Clinical Trials. Biomed Res Int. 2017; 2017:2356346. doi: 10.1155/2017/2356346. Epub 2017 Sep 20. PMID: 29291206; PMCID: PMC5632473.

14. Li JX, Hong Y, Chan KM. Tai Chi: physiological characteristics and beneficial effects on health. Br J Sports Med. (2001) 35:148–56. doi: 10.1136/bjsm.35.3.148

15. Wolf SL, Sattin RW, Kutner M, O'Grady M, Greenspan AI, Gregor RJ. Intense Tai Chi exercise training and fall occurrences in older, transitionally frail adults: a randomized, controlled trial. J Am Geriatr Soc. (2003) 51:1693–701. doi: 10.1046/j.1532-5415.2003. 51552.x

16. Li F, Harmer P, Fitzgerald K, Eckstrom E, Stock R, Galver J, et al. Tai Chi and postural stability in patients with Parkinson's disease. N Engl J Med. (2012) 366:511–9. doi: 10.1056/NEJMoa1107911

17. Wang C, Schmid CH, Fielding RA, Harvey WF, Reid KF, Price LL, Driban JB, Kalish R, Rones R, McAlindon T. Effect of tai chi versus aerobic exercise for fibromyalgia: comparative effectiveness randomized controlled trial. BMJ. 2018 Mar 21;360: k851. doi: 10.1136/bmj. k851. PMID: 29563100; PMCID: PMC5861462.

18. Wang X, Luo H. Effects of traditional Chinese exercise therapy on pain scores, sleep quality, and anxiety-depression symptoms in fibromyalgia patients: a systematic review and meta-analysis. BMC Musculoskelet Disord. 2024 Jan 27;25(1):99. Doi: 10.1186/s12891-024-07194-7. PMID: 38281020; PMCID: PMC10821260.

19. Zamunér AR, Andrade CP, Arca EA, Avila MA. Impact of water therapy on pain management in patients with fibromyalgia: current perspectives. J Pain Res. 2019 Jul 3; 12:1971-2007. doi: 10.2147/JPR.S161494. PMID: 31308729; PMCID: PMC6613198.

20. Bravo C, Rubí-Carnacea F, Colomo I, Sánchez-de-la-Torre M, Fernández-Lago H, Climent-Sanz C. Aquatic therapy improves self-reported sleep quality in fibromyalgia patients: a systematic review and meta-analysis. Sleep Breath. 2024 May;28(2):565-583. doi: 10.1007/s11325-023-02933-x. Epub 2023 Oct 17. PMID: 37847348; PMCID: PMC11136798.

21. Barker AL, Talevski J, Morello RT, Brand CA, Rahmann AE, Urquhart DM. Effectiveness of aquatic exercise for musculoskeletal conditions: a meta-analysis. Arch Phys Med Rehabil. 2014 Sep;95(9):1776-86. doi: 10.1016/j.apmr.2014.04.005. Epub 2014 Apr 24. PMID: 24769068.

22. Lima TB, Dias JM, Mazuquin BF, da Silva CT, Nogueira RM, Marques AP, Lavado EL, Cardoso JR. The effectiveness of aquatic physical therapy in the treatment of fibromyalgia: a systematic review with meta-analysis. Clin Rehabil. 2013 Oct;27(10):892-908. doi: 10.1177/0269215513484772. Epub 2013 Jul 1. PMID: 23818412.

23. Choy EH. The role of sleep in pain and fibromyalgia. Nat Rev Rheumatol. 2015 Sep;11(9):513-20. doi: 10.1038/nrrheum.2015.56. Epub 2015 Apr 28. PMID: 25907704.

24. Nelson KL, Davis JE, Corbett CF. Sleep quality: An evolutionary concept analysis. Nurs Forum. 2022 Jan;57(1):144-151. Doi: 10.1111/nuf.12659. Epub 2021 Oct 5. PMID: 34610163.

25. Poole JL, Siegel P. Effectiveness of Occupational Therapy Interventions for Adults With Fibromyalgia: A Systematic Review. Am J Occup Ther. 2017 Jan/Feb;71(1):7101180040p1-7101180040p10. doi: 10.5014/ajot.2017.023192. PMID: 28027041.

26. Siegel P, Jones BL, Poole JL. Occupational Therapy Interventions for Adults With Fibromyalgia. Am J Occup Ther. 2018 Sep/Oct;72(5):7205395010p1-7205395010p4. doi: 10.5014/ajot.2018.725002. PMID: 30157022.

27. Johnson M. Transcutaneous Electrical Nerve Stimulation: Mechanisms, Clinical Application and Evidence. Rev Pain. 2007 Aug;1(1):7-11. doi: 10.1177/204946370700100103. PMID: 26526976; PMCID: PMC4589923.

28. Johnson MI, Bjordal JM. Transcutaneous electrical nerve stimulation for the management of painful conditions: focus on neuropathic pain. Expert Rev Neurother. 2011 May;11(5):735-53. doi: 10.1586/ern.11.48. PMID: 21539490.

29. Johnson MI, Claydon LS, Herbison GP, Jones G, Paley CA. Transcutaneous electrical nerve stimulation (TENS) for fibromyalgia in adults. Cochrane Database Syst Rev. 2017 Oct 9;10(10): CD012172. Doi: 10.1002/14651858.CD012172.pub2. PMID: 28990665; PMCID: PMC6485914.

30. Dailey DL, Rakel BA, Vance CGT, Liebano RE, Amrit AS, Bush HM, Lee KS, Lee JE, Sluka KA. Transcutaneous electrical nerve stimulation reduces pain, fatigue, and hyperalgesia while restoring central inhibition in primary fibromyalgia. Pain. 2013 Nov;154(11):2554-2562. doi: 10.1016/j.pain.2013.07.043. Epub 2013 Jul 27. PMID: 23900134; PMCID: PMC3972497.

31. Gur A. Physical therapy modalities in the management of fibromyalgia. Curr Pharm Des. 2006;12(1):29-35. PMID: 16454722.

32. NIH Consensus Conference. Acupuncture. JAMA. 1998 Nov 4;280(17):1518-24. PMID: 9809733

33. Waylonis GW. Long-term follow-up on patients with fibrositis treated with acupuncture. Ohio State Med J. 1977 May;73(5):299-302. PMID: 266143.

34. Sprott H, Jeschonneck M, Grohmann G, Heim G. Microcirculatory changes over the tender points in fibromyalgia patients after acupuncture therapy (measured with laser-doppler flowmetry). Wien Klin Wochenschr 2000; 112: 580-86.

35. Targino RA, Imamura MHS, Kaziyama HHS, Souza LP, Hsing WT, Imamura ST. Pain treatment with acupuncture for patients with fibromyalgia. Curr Pain Headache Rep 2002; 6: 379-83.

36. Panton L, Simonavice E, Williams K, Mojock C, Kim JS, Kingsley JD, McMillan V, Mathis R. Effects of Class IV laser therapy on fibromyalgia impact and function in women with fibromyalgia. J Altern Complement Med. 2013 May;19(5):445-52. doi: 10.1089/acm.2011.0398. Epub 2012 Nov 23. PMID: 23176373.

37. Dos Santos RC, Souza Guedes KWHS, de Sousa Pinto JM, Oliveira MF. Acute low-level laser therapy effects on peripheral muscle strength and resistance in patients with fibromyalgia. Lasers Med Sci. 2020 Mar;35(2):505-510. doi: 10.1007/s10103-019-02816-2. Epub 2019 Jun 5. PMID: 31165945.

38. Gür A, Karakoç M, Nas K, Cevik R, Saraç J, Demir E. Efficacy of low power laser therapy in fibromyalgia: a single-blind, placebo-controlled trial. Lasers Med Sci. 2002;17(1):57-61. doi: 10.1007/s10103-002-8267-4. PMID: 11845369.

39. Chipon E, Bosson JL, Minier L, Dumolard A, Vilotitch A, Crouzier D, Maindet C. A drug-free solution for improving the quality of life of fibromyalgia patients (Fibrepik): study protocol of a multicenter, randomized, controlled effectiveness trial. Trials. 2022 Sep 5;23(1):740. doi: 10.1186/s13063-022-06693-z. PMID: 36064731; PMCID: PMC9442919.

40. Paolucci T, Piccinini G, Iosa M, Piermattei C, de Angelis S, Grasso MR, Zangrando F, Saraceni VM. Efficacy of extremely low-frequency magnetic field in fibromyalgia pain: A pilot study. J Rehabil Res Dev. 2016;53(6):1023-1034. doi: 10.1682/JRRD.2015.04.0061. PMID: 28475205.

41. Bennett R, Nelson D. Cognitive behavioral therapy for fibromyalgia. Nat Clin Pract Rheumatol. 2006 Aug;2(8):416-24. doi: 10.1038/ncprheum0245. PMID: 16932733.

42. Vallejo MA, Ortega J, Rivera J, Comeche MI, Vallejo-Slocker L. Internet versus face-to-face group cognitive-behavioral therapy for fibromyalgia: A randomized control trial. J Psychiatr Res. 2015 Sep; 68:106-13. doi: 10.1016/j.jpsychires.2015.06.006. Epub 2015 Jun 20. PMID: 26228408.

43. Turk DC, Monarch ES, Williams AD. Psychological evaluation of patients diagnosed with fibromyalgia syndrome: a comprehensive approach. Rheum Dis Clin North Am. 2002 May;28(2):219-33. doi: 10.1016/s0889-857x(01)00003-5. PMID: 12122915

44. Goldenberg DL, Burckhardt C, Crofford L. Management of fibromyalgia syndrome. JAMA. 2004 Nov 17;292(19):2388-95. doi: 10.1001/jama.292.19.2388. PMID: 15547167.

45. Fonia D, Aisenberg D. The Effects of Mindfulness Interventions on Fibromyalgia in Adults aged 65 and Older: A Window to Effective Therapy. J Clin Psychol Med Settings. 2023 Sep;30(3):543-560. doi: 10.1007/s10880-022-09911-7. Epub 2022 Sep 26. PMID: 36163446.

46. Morone NE, Rollman BL, Moore CG, Li Q, Weiner DK. A mind-body program for older adults with chronic low back pain: results of a pilot study. Pain Med. 2009 Nov;10(8):1395-407. doi: 10.1111/j.1526-4637.2009.00746. x. PMID: 20021599; PMCID: PMC2849802.

47. Parra-Delgado, M., & Latorre-Postigo, J. M. (2013). Effectiveness of mindfulness-based cognitive therapy in the treatment of fibromyalgia: A randomized trial. Cognitive Therapy and Research, 37(5), 1015–1026. https://doi.org/10.1007/s10608-013-9538-z

48. Schmidt S, Grossman P, Schwarzer B, Jena S, Naumann J, Walach H. Treating fibromyalgia with mindfulness-based stress reduction: results from a 3-armed randomized controlled trial. Pain. 2011 Feb;152(2):361-369. doi: 10.1016/j.pain.2010.10.043. Epub 2010 Dec 13. PMID: 21146930.

49. Tomas-Carus P, Branco JC, Raimundo A, Parra JA, Batalha N, Biehl-Printes C. Breathing Exercises Must Be a Real and Effective Intervention to Consider in Women with Fibromyalgia: A Pilot Randomized Controlled Trial. J Altern Complement Med. 2018 Aug;24(8):825-832. doi: 10.1089/acm.2017.0335. Epub 2018 Apr 13. PMID: 29653069.

50. Rossi A, Di Lollo AC, Guzzo MP, Giacomelli C, Atzeni F, Bazzichi L, Di Franco M. Fibromyalgia and nutrition: what news? Clin Exp Rheumatol. 2015 Jan-Feb;33(1 Suppl 88):S117-25. Epub 2015 Mar 18. PMID: 25786053.

51. Bjørklund G, Dadar M, Chirumbolo S, Aaseth J. Fibromyalgia and nutrition: Therapeutic possibilities? Biomed Pharmacother. 2018 Jul; 103:531-538. doi 10.1016/j.biopha.2018.04.056. Epub 2018 Apr 24. PMID: 29677539.

Nutrition and Fibromyalgia

Clara Nemr

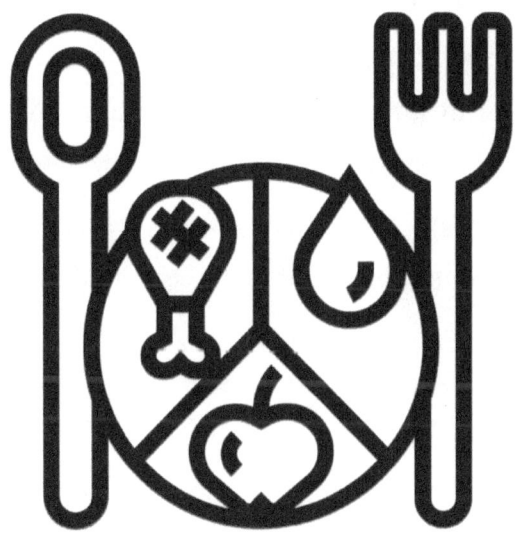

Introduction

Fibromyalgia (FM) is a complex chronic pain disorder that affects millions of people worldwide, causing widespread musculoskeletal pain, fatigue, and other symptoms. While the exact cause remains unknown, research has increasingly focused on the potential role of nutrition in managing fibromyalgia symptoms. Certain nutrients and dietary approaches have shown promise in alleviating pain, reducing inflammation, and improving the overall quality of life for those with fibromyalgia.

Nutrition is widely recognized as crucial in disease prevention, with the World Health Nutrition Organization supporting dietary measures to prevent chronic illnesses. Recent research emphasizes nutrition's role in treating FM, spotlighting antioxidants' benefits in reducing oxidative stress. High BMI, nutritional deficiencies, imbalanced diets, and certain food additives may exacerbate FM symptoms, suggesting that modified diets could be a therapeutic option[1].

Vitamin Deficiencies

Nutritional status plays a crucial role in the management of fibromyalgia (FM), with recent research focusing on the impact of vitamin deficiencies on symptom severity. FM has been associated with deficiencies in vitamins A, D, and E. A study showed that FM patients showed significantly lower levels of vitamins A, E, and D ($p < 0,001$) and higher lipid peroxidation (LP) levels compared to controls. These findings suggest a possible link between fat-soluble antioxidants, oxidative stress, and FM[2]. Additionally, obesity may worsen vitamin D deficiency by trapping the vitamin in fat tissue.

Studies show that patients with low vitamin D levels (<30 ng/ml) report higher pain scores on the Visual Analog Scale (VAS) compared to those with normal levels [3]. These insights highlight the importance of addressing vitamin deficiencies, particularly in fat-soluble vitamins, as part of a comprehensive approach to FM management.

Supplementation

The World Health Organization recognizes diet as a "modifiable determinant" of pain, suggesting that chronic musculoskeletal pain may have nutritional factors beyond psychological and cognitive aspects. Essential fatty acids like eicosapentaenoic acids, arachidonic acids, and tryptophan have shown pain-relieving effects in the central nervous system[4]. The direct correlation between vitamins and nutritional supplements and the pathophysiology of chronic pain remains disputed, with some studies finding no significant benefit from supplementation[5]. However, there are mechanisms by which vitamin D may be beneficial in FM.

Vitamin D plays a crucial role in various physiological processes related to pain perception and inflammation. It modulates nociceptive transmission in skeletal muscles, and its deficiency may result in hyperinnervation and increased sensitivity to musculoskeletal pain[6]. Additionally, vitamin D exhibits anti-inflammatory and immunomodulatory properties, notably by reducing the production of prostaglandin E2, which helps regulate inflammatory pathways. Furthermore, this vitamin influences the synthesis and functioning of neurotransmitters, including serotonin, which is known to be altered in fibromyalgia (FM) patients. These diverse effects of vitamin D highlight its potential importance in managing FM symptoms and understanding the underlying mechanisms of the condition[7].

Observational studies have suggested a potential connection between vitamin D deficiency and chronic pain, particularly in fibromyalgia (FM). Vitamin D deficiency may also play a role in central sensitization, and several studies have confirmed its involvement in chronic musculoskeletal pain. A double-blind, placebo-controlled study was conducted with 30 participants (27 women, three men) who met the American College of Rheumatology criteria for FM and had serum calcifediol levels below 80 nmol/L. The treatment group received daily doses of cholecalciferol (vitamin D3) based on their initial serum calcifediol levels to maintain levels between 80 and 120 nmol/L. The placebo group received a triglyceride solution without cholecalciferol. The results of this study demonstrated a significant reduction in mean scores on the Visual Analog Scale (VAS) for pain in the treatment group, suggesting that vitamin D supplementation may be beneficial for FM patients with vitamin D deficiency[8].

Vitamin B12 has several beneficial effects on pain management. It inhibits inflammatory mediators that contribute to pain, thereby potentially reducing inflammation-related discomfort. Additionally, vitamin B12 enhances the effectiveness of norepinephrine and 5-hydroxytryptamine as inhibitory signals in the pain pathway, leading to a decrease in pain perception. Furthermore, it promotes the regeneration of damaged nerves and inhibits spontaneous ectopic neuronal activity, which is associated with unnecessary pain and increased sensitivity to pain. These combined actions suggest that vitamin B12 can play a significant role in alleviating various types of pain, particularly those related to inflammation and nerve damage[7]. Clinical studies have demonstrated the potential benefits of vitamin B12 in treating fibromyalgia (FM). One study found that FM patients who received regular B12 injections along with oral B9 supplements experienced symptom relief. However, the treatment was less effective for those using opioids for pain management and more effective for patients taking thyroid hormones for hypothyroidism. Another study showed that daily administration of 1000 µg of oral vitamin B12 for 50 days significantly improved the severity of FM symptoms and anxiety scores in patients[9].

Similarly, Magnesium can alleviate inflammation and pain associated with fibromyalgia (FM) symptoms. Individuals with FM often have low magnesium levels, which can reduce exercise capacity, increase inflammation, and cause muscle spasms. Magnesium is crucial for muscle relaxation and neurotransmitter functions, playing a key role in preventing central sensitization—a primary mechanism underlying FM. It blocks N-methyl-D-aspartate (NMDA) receptors in a voltage-dependent manner, thus preventing central sensitization[10].

Magnesium deficiency is linked to common FM symptoms such as muscle pain, fatigue, sleep difficulties, and anxiety. This is due to magnesium's role in muscle function regulation and adenosine triphosphate (ATP) production, as ATP is stored in the body as a magnesium-ATP compound[11]. Low ATP levels, common in FM patients, are thought to contribute significantly to symptom development. Furthermore, magnesium is involved in hormone synthesis regulation, including norepinephrine, which is often overproduced in FM patients and contributes to the condition's pathogenesis. Magnesium also regulates various nerve receptors, such as NMDA and 5-HT3, which are involved in neuropathic pain. By blocking these receptors, magnesium may help alleviate some types of FM pain[12].

Prebiotic and probiotic supplements have been shown to reduce pain symptoms in patients with FM. Recent research suggests that gut microorganisms influence brain processes, affecting pain, depression, and sleep. A clinical trial investigated the effects of probiotics and prebiotics on fibromyalgia syndrome symptoms in 53 female participants. The 8-week study compared probiotic, prebiotic, and placebo treatments. Results showed probiotics significantly improved depression, anxiety, sleep quality, and pain scores, while prebiotics improved sleep quality and pain scores. The study supports the potential use of probiotics in managing FM symptoms, offering a promising treatment strategy[13].

Omega-3 fatty acids, particularly EPA and DHA, play a crucial role in managing fibromyalgia (FM) through their anti-inflammatory properties. These fatty acids and their derivatives (resolvins, maresins, and protectins) target neuroinflammation, a key factor in FM, by stimulating the cessation of inflammation in immune cells[14]. This action helps disrupt the cycle of neuroinflammation associated with FM.

Additionally, a balanced intake of saturated and unsaturated fats, including omega-3 and omega-6, may influence endocannabinoid production, contributing to pain relief. Studies have shown that omega-3 fatty acids can reduce pain intensity and fatigue while improving sleep quality in FM patients[15]. A study by Del Giorno et al. in 2015 investigated the effectiveness of combining duloxetine (DLX) and pregabalin (PGB) for treating fibromyalgia (FM) syndrome. The research also explored the potential added benefits of including palmitoylethanolamide (PEA), a lipid signaling molecule, in the treatment regimen. The results demonstrated that the DLX + PGB combination reduced both the number of pain points and pain intensity in FM patients after 3 and 6 months of treatment. Furthermore, when PEA was added to the DLX + PGB combination, patients experienced an even more significant improvement in pain symptoms compared to those receiving only DLX + PGB[16]. This study suggests that combination therapy using DLX and PGB can be effective in managing FM symptoms and that adding PEA to this combination may provide additional pain relief for FM patients.

Acetyl-L-carnitine (ALA) has demonstrated potential as a treatment for FM due to several mechanisms of action. Firstly, ALA modulates neurotransmitters such as acetylcholine, serotonin, and dopamine, which play crucial roles in pain perception and mood regulation[17]. This modulation suggests that ALA could help alleviate the cognitive and mood disorders often associated with FM.

Additionally, ALA targets neurotrophic factors like nerve growth factor and metabotropic glutamate receptors through epigenetic mechanisms, further supporting its therapeutic potential[18]. Moreover, ALA possesses antioxidant properties that protect against oxidative stress, which is significant considering the possible involvement of mitochondrial dysfunction and neuroinflammation in the pathogenesis of FM[19]. In a randomized controlled trial, the combination of ALA with the antidepressant duloxetine and the anticonvulsant pregabalin was shown to effectively treat FM symptoms. This combination therapy resulted in significant improvements in pain, fatigue, sleep, and depression compared to the use of duloxetine and pregabalin alone[18].

S-adenosylmethionine (SAMe) is a naturally occurring compound crucial for various cellular processes, including methylation reactions, transsulfuration, and aminopropylation. In fibromyalgia (FM), SAMe has shown potential therapeutic benefits through multiple mechanisms.

It plays a key role in methylation and gene expression, particularly in pain signaling pathways, addressing altered methylation patterns observed in FM[20]. SAMe modulates pain transmission by influencing neurotransmitters like serotonin and dopamine, potentially reducing pain perception. Its anti-inflammatory properties may alleviate symptoms such as pain, fatigue, and stiffness[21]. Additionally, SAMe's neuroprotective qualities could help counteract neurodegenerative changes associated with FM[20]. Finally, SAMe may exhibit synergistic effects when combined with other treatments, enhancing its therapeutic potential in FM management.

Curcumin, the active compound in turmeric, has shown potential benefits for treating fibromyalgia (FM) symptoms due to its anti-inflammatory and antioxidant properties. One of the mechanisms by which curcumin exerts its effects is by decreasing the production of pro-inflammatory cytokines[22]. Specifically, curcumin can inhibit the production of interleukin-12 (IL-12) by CD4, CD8, and natural killer (NK) cells, thereby reducing inflammation[23]. Additionally, curcumin enhances the body's antioxidant capacity by increasing the levels of antioxidant enzymes such as catalase, superoxide dismutase, and glutathione in the nervous system, skeletal muscles, and circulatory system, which helps mitigate oxidative stress[24]. Furthermore, curcumin may modulate neuroinflammation by reducing the release of inflammatory mediators from spinal glial cells, including microglia and astrocytes, which can decrease neuronal excitability and improve chronic pain[19]. These mechanisms collectively highlight curcumin's potential as a natural therapeutic agent for managing FM symptoms.

Melatonin has been utilized in neurology and various pain syndromes, including fibromyalgia (FM). As a potent endogenous antioxidant, melatonin regulates circadian rhythms, pain modulation, mood, and immune balance. In FM treatment, melatonin has demonstrated efficacy in improving sleep quality, pain levels, and pain thresholds by enhancing the descending endogenous pain-modulating system[25]. The mechanism of action involves decreased melatonin nuclear receptor expression and enhanced cytokine production in lymphocytic and monocytic cell lines, indicating anti-inflammatory effects. Melatonin's analgesic properties are mediated through activation of supraspinal sites, inhibition of spinal nociception, and modulation of GABAergic, opioid, and glutamatergic systems[26]. Given its ability to affect multiple pathways involved in FM pathophysiology, melatonin is considered a promising adjunctive treatment for this chronic pain syndrome. Its multifaceted approach to addressing various aspects of FM makes it a valuable component in managing the condition[27].

Coenzyme Q10 (CoQ10) is essential for the electron transport chain in mitochondria, aiding in the generation of adenosine triphosphate (ATP), the primary energy source for cells. In FM, there is a reduction in mitochondrial mass and CoQ10 levels, which results in decreased energy production and heightened oxidative stress[28]. CoQ10 is a potent antioxidant that shields cells from oxidative damage caused by reactive oxygen species (ROS). In FM, excessive ROS can lead to pain and inflammation, so CoQ10's antioxidant properties help alleviate these symptoms[29]. Additionally, CoQ10 influences gene expression, particularly genes associated with chronic inflammation, and exhibits anti-inflammatory effects, indicating its potential to reduce inflammation in FM[30]. While research is still preliminary, CoQ10 appears promising in alleviating both pain and anxiety in FM patients.

Gluten Sensitivity in Fibromyalgia

The relationship between diet and FM symptoms has been a subject of increasing interest in recent years, with particular attention given to gluten sensitivity. Research suggests a higher prevalence of food allergies or intolerances in FM patients. Studies on gluten-free diets for FM due to common gluten sensitivity showed promising results. In one study of 246 patients on a 3-month gluten-free diet, 36% responded positively, with 8% experiencing significant improvements in FM symptoms, gastrointestinal issues, pain, and fatigue[31]. These findings highlight the potential benefits of dietary modifications, particularly gluten elimination, in managing FM symptoms for some patients, though more research is needed to fully understand the mechanisms and long-term effects of such interventions.

Foods to Avoid

Considering foods to avoid for Fibromyalgia (FM), recent research has focused on the relationship between neurochemicals, neurohormones, and nutrition in the pathophysiology of FM. Particular attention has been given to the role of certain amino acids and neurotransmitters, specifically glutamate and aspartate, which are found in common food additives. These compounds, while essential for normal neurotransmission, can potentially become excitotoxic in excessive amounts, leading to neuronal damage[32].

Several studies have investigated the effects of eliminating monosodium glutamate (MSG) and aspartame from the diets of FM patients. Some research has shown improvement in FM symptoms following the removal of these additives from patients' diets. For instance, one study reported symptom improvement one month after eliminating MSG and aspartame, although these benefits were not sustained at the three-month mark[33].

The potential link between dietary glutamate and aspartate and neurotransmission regulation in FM patients suggests that avoiding foods containing these additives may be beneficial. Common sources of MSG include processed foods, canned vegetables, soups, and Chinese cuisine, while aspartame is frequently found in diet sodas and sugar-free products. Given that eliminating these additives from one's diet poses minimal risk and offers potential benefits, it may be worth considering for FM patients[34].

However, it's important to note that more comprehensive, long-term studies with larger sample sizes are needed to definitively establish the efficacy of this dietary approach. While the current evidence is promising, it remains inconclusive, and individual responses may vary. FM patients considering dietary changes should consult with their healthcare providers to ensure a balanced and nutritionally adequate diet while exploring potential symptom management strategies.

Dietary Interventions

Dietary interventions have shown promising results in managing fibromyalgia (FM) symptoms, with various studies exploring the impact of different dietary approaches on patient outcomes.

A study conducted on 84 outpatients with fibromyalgia, involving clinical, nutritional, and dietary assessments, showed that the participants in the personalized Mediterranean diet group showed improvements in various FM parameters such as disability scores, fatigue, and anxiety compared to the no-diet group. The results revealed that most patients had poor eating habits, including inadequate food choices, improper meal timing, and unbalanced nutrient composition.

The study concluded that consuming inflammatory foods or meals with incorrect nutritional content may exacerbate the condition of FM patients. Paying proper attention to eating habits could lead to an improved quality of life for individuals with FM[35].

Another study was conducted on 45 female FM patients, comparing the effects of two different diets over 45 days: the holoprotein diet, characterized by minimal carbohydrate intake with tailored protein and lipid quantities, and the LOGI diet, which includes moderate levels of low-glycemic-index carbohydrates. Both diets improved FM symptoms, but the holoprotein diet showed more pronounced effects. NMR analysis revealed distinct changes in metabolic profiles corresponding to symptom improvements. The LOGI diet primarily impacted energy metabolism, while the holoprotein diet induced more systemic changes, potentially affecting metabolic pathways related to FM dysfunction. Although further research is needed, these findings suggest that the holoprotein diet could be an effective treatment for significantly reducing FM symptoms. In contrast, the LOGI diet may be beneficial for maintaining the improvements achieved with the holoprotein diet over time[36].

Similarly, a study on 23 women with fibromyalgia (FM) found that consuming 50 mL of organic olive oil daily for 3 weeks may protect against oxidative stress and improve functional capacity and psychological status. Biochemical analyses showed increased antioxidant compounds and enzyme activities. After 3 weeks, significant reductions in oxidative damage markers were observed, suggesting that extra virgin olive oil may help reduce oxidative stress in women with FM[37]. These studies highlight the potential of tailored dietary interventions in managing FM symptoms and improving patients' quality of life. Further research is needed to establish standardized dietary guidelines for FM patients and to understand the long-term effects of these interventions.

Recent studies indicate that vegetarian and vegan diets can effectively manage fibromyalgia (FM) due to their anti-inflammatory effects on the gut microbiome and overall systemic inflammation. Meta-analyses show that these diets are associated with lower C-reactive protein levels compared to omnivorous diets, suggesting a reduced risk of chronic diseases. Vegetarians typically consume grains, fruits, vegetables, legumes, and nuts, which have been studied for their health benefits, though there is no consensus on their anti-inflammatory effects. The anti-inflammatory impact of these diets varies depending on the specific foods consumed, with phytosterols being particularly potent in reducing inflammation[38].

Other research highlighted the benefits of a vegetarian diet in FM patients, emphasizing increased vitamin A intake from carrot juice and the inclusion of fresh fruits, salads, raw vegetables, nuts, seeds, whole grains, tubers, flaxseed oil, and extra virgin olive oil while avoiding alcohol, caffeine, refined sugar, corn syrup, refined oils, flour, dairy, eggs, and meat. This diet improved FM symptoms in 19 out of 30 participants, as measured by self-reported questionnaires [39].

A systematic review of six studies, including four clinical trials and two cohort studies, found significant improvements in quality of life, pain, sleep quality, anxiety, depression, and general health for FM patients on a vegetarian diet. The review suggests that physical exercise and maintaining an energy deficit are also important, as higher BMI levels are linked to increased pain and functional issues in FM patients[40].

Exercise

The complementary effect of exercise and nutrition in treating fibromyalgia (FM) symptoms is achieved by combining low-impact aerobic exercise with a balanced diet. Studies have demonstrated that regular aerobic activities like walking, swimming, or cycling can improve fitness, reduce pain and fatigue, and enhance daily functioning in FM patients[41]. Research indicates that exercise is crucial for maintaining muscle strength, flexibility, weight control, and overall well-being, potentially altering levels of endorphins and serotonin, which affect pain threshold, mood, and anxiety. A study aiming to assess the effectiveness of a multidisciplinary intervention based on nutrition, chronobiology, and physical exercise in improving lifestyle and quality of life for individuals with FM and chronic fatigue syndrome (CFS) employs a mixed-methods approach, including a randomized clinical trial and qualitative analysis. Participants were divided into a control group receiving usual care and an intervention group receiving an additional 12-hour program over four days. The study found that the intervention improved symptoms such as pain, fatigue, and insomnia, as well as enhanced food and exercise habits, ultimately leading to better quality of life and reduced healthcare costs [42].

To maximize this combined effect, a collaborative approach involving various healthcare professionals is necessary, considering individual patient comorbidities. Recent meta-analyses have compared the effectiveness of different physical and dietary interventions. A 2022 study evaluated acupuncture, intravenous lidocaine, diet, physiotherapy, and placebo in FM patients. Acupuncture showed the most significant improvements in quality of life, pain, and depression levels compared to placebo. Physiotherapy also demonstrated notable benefits in quality of life. However, lidocaine and diet alone did not show significant differences compared to placebo[43].

Conclusion

The relationship between nutrition and fibromyalgia is increasingly recognized as a critical area of research and clinical practice. This study highlights the significant role of nutrition in managing fibromyalgia (FM) symptoms and improving patients' quality of life. Various nutrients, including vitamins D, B12, and magnesium, as well as dietary interventions such as the Mediterranean diet, gluten-free diet, and vegetarian/vegan diets, have shown promise in alleviating pain, reducing inflammation, and enhancing overall well-being. The findings underscore the importance of addressing nutritional deficiencies and adopting tailored dietary approaches as part of a comprehensive treatment plan for FM. Additionally, the combination of proper nutrition with physical exercise appears to be particularly effective in managing FM symptoms. While these results are promising, further research is needed to establish standardized dietary guidelines and understand the long-term effects of these interventions. A multidisciplinary approach, incorporating personalized nutritional advice and other therapeutic strategies, is essential for optimizing the management of FM and improving patients' quality of life. By focusing on personalized and evidence-based dietary modifications, healthcare providers can offer FM patients a promising pathway to better health and symptom relief.

References:

1. Kadayifci FZ, Bradley MJ, Onat AM, Shi HN, Zheng S (2022) Review of nutritional approaches to fibromyalgia. Nutrition Reviews 80:2260–2274. https://doi.org/10.1093/nutrit/nuac036

2. Akkuş S, Nazıroğlu M, Eriş S, Yalman K, Yılmaz N, Yener M (2009) Levels of lipid peroxidation, nitric oxide, and antioxidant vitamins in plasma of patients with fibromyalgia. Cell Biochemistry & Function 27:181–185. https://doi.org/10.1002/cbf.1548

3. Chang K-V (2015) Is Serum Hypovitaminosis D Associatedwith Chronic Widespread Pain IncludingFibromyalgia? A Meta-analysis of ObservationalStudies. Pain Phys 5;18:E877–E887. https://doi.org/10.36076/ppj.2015/18/E877

4. Elma Ö, Yilmaz ST, Deliens T, Coppieters I, Clarys P, Nijs J, Malfliet A (2020) Do Nutritional Factors Interact with Chronic Musculoskeletal Pain? A Systematic Review. JCM 9:702. https://doi.org/10.3390/jcm9030702

5. Kurapatti M, Carreira D (2023) Diet Composition's Effect on Chronic Musculoskeletal Pain: A Narrative Review. Pain Physician 26:527–534

6. Sarzi-Puttini P, Giorgi V, Atzeni F, Gorla R, Kosek E, Choy EH, Bazzichi L, Häuser W, Ablin JN, Aloush V, Buskila D, Amital H, Da Silva JAP, Perrot S, Morlion B, Polati E, Schweiger V, Coaccioli S, Varrassi G, Di Franco M, Torta R, Øien Forseth KM, Mannerkorpi K, Salaffi F, Di Carlo M, Cassisi G, Batticciotto A (2021) Diagnostic and therapeutic care pathway for fibromyalgia. Clinical and Experimental Rheumatology 39:120–127.

https://doi.org/10.55563/clinexprheumatol/zcp5hz

7. Haddad HW, Mallepalli NR, Scheinuk JE, Bhargava P, Cornett EM, Urits I, Kaye AD (2021) The Role of Nutrient Supplementation in the Management of Chronic Pain in Fibromyalgia: A Narrative Review. Pain Ther 10:827–848. https://doi.org/10.1007/s40122-021-00266-9

8. Wepner F, Scheuer R, Schuetz-Wieser B, Machacek P, Pieler-Bruha E, Cross HS, Hahne J, Friedrich M (2014) Effects of vitamin D on patients with fibromyalgia syndrome: A randomized placebo-controlled trial. Pain 155:261–268. https://doi.org/10.1016/j.pain.2013.10.002

9. Gharibpoor F, Ghavidel-Parsa B, Sattari N, Bidari A, Nejatifar F, Montazeri A (2022) Effect of vitamin B12 on the symptom severity and psychological profile of fibromyalgia patients; a prospective pre-post study. BMC Rheumatol 6:51. https://doi.org/10.1186/s41927-022-00282-y

10. Kim Y-S, Kim K-M, Lee D-J, Kim B-T, Park S-B, Cho D-Y, Suh C-H, Kim H-A, Park R-W, Joo N-S (2011) Women with Fibromyalgia Have Lower Levels of Calcium, Magnesium, Iron and Manganese in Hair Mineral Analysis. J Korean Med Sci 26:1253. https://doi.org/10.3346/jkms.2011.26.10.1253

11. Boulis M, Boulis M, Clauw D (2021) Magnesium and Fibromyalgia: A Literature Review. J Prim Care Community Health 12:21501327211038. https://doi.org/10.1177/21501327211038433

12. Macian N, Dualé C, Voute M, Leray V, Courrent M, Bodé P, Giron F, Sonneville S, Bernard L, Joanny F, Menard K, Ducheix G, Pereira B, Pickering G (2022) Short-Term Magnesium Therapy Alleviates Moderate Stress in Patients with Fibromyalgia: A Randomized Double-Blind Clinical Trial. Nutrients 14:2088.

https://doi.org/10.3390/nu14102088

13. Aslan Çİn NN, Açik M, Tertemİz OF, Aktan Ç, Akçali DT, Çakiroğlu FP, Özçelİk AÖ (2024) Effect of prebiotic and probiotic supplementation on reduced pain in patients with fibromyalgia syndrome: a double-blind, placebo-controlled randomized clinical trial. Psychology, Health & Medicine 29:528–541. https://doi.org/10.1080/13548506.2023.2216464

14. Herbst EAF, Paglialunga S, Gerling C, Whitfield J, Mukai K, Chabowski A, Heigenhauser GJF, Spriet LL, Holloway GP (2014) Omega-3 supplementation alters mitochondrial membrane composition and respiration kinetics in human skeletal muscle. The Journal of Physiology 592:1341–1352. https://doi.org/10.1113/jphysiol.2013.267336

15. Bourke SL, Schlag AK, O'Sullivan SE, Nutt DJ, Finn DP (2022) Cannabinoids and the endocannabinoid system in fibromyalgia: A review of preclinical and clinical research. Pharmacology & Therapeutics 240:108216. https://doi.org/10.1016/j.pharmthera.2022.108216

16. Del Giorno R, Skaper S, Paladini A, Varrassi G, Coaccioli S (2015) Palmitoylethanolamide in Fibromyalgia: Results from Prospective and Retrospective Observational Studies. Pain Ther 4:169–178. https://doi.org/10.1007/s40122-015-0038-6

17. Saracoglu I, Akin E, Aydin Dincer GB (2022) Efficacy of adding pain neuroscience education to a multimodal treatment in fibromyalgia: A systematic review and meta-analysis. Int J of Rheum Dis 25:394–404. https://doi.org/10.1111/1756-185X.14293

18. Rossini M, Di Munno O, Valentini G, Bianchi G, Biasi G, Cacace E, Malesci D, La Montagna G, Viapiana O, Adami S (2007) Double-blind, multicenter trial comparing acetyl l-carnitine with placebo in the treatment of fibromyalgia patients. Clin Exp Rheumatol 25:182–188

19. Sarzi-Puttini P, Giorgi V, Di Lascio S, Fornasari D (2021) Acetyl-L-carnitine in chronic pain: A narrative review. Pharmacological Research 173:105874. https://doi.org/10.1016/j.phrs.2021.105874

20. Gerra MC, Carnevali D, Ossola P, González-Villar A, Pedersen IS, Triñanes Y, Donnini C, Manfredini M, Arendt-Nielsen L, Carrillo-de-la-Peña MT (2021) DNA Methylation Changes in Fibromyalgia Suggest the Role of the Immune-Inflammatory Response and Central Sensitization. JCM 10:4992. https://doi.org/10.3390/jcm10214992

21. Pfalzer AC, Choi S-W, Tammen SA, Park LK, Bottiglieri T, Parnell LD, Lamon-Fava S (2014) S-adenosylmethionine mediates inhibition of inflammatory response and changes in DNA methylation in human macrophages. Physiological Genomics 46:617–623. https://doi.org/10.1152/physiolgenomics.00056.2014

22. Hasriadi, Dasuni Wasana PW, Vajragupta O, Rojsitthisak P, Towiwat P (2021) Mechanistic Insight into the Effects of Curcumin on Neuroinflammation-Driven Chronic Pain. Pharmaceuticals 14:777. https://doi.org/10.3390/ph14080777

23. Shen C-L, Schuck A, Tompkins C, Dunn DM, Neugebauer V (2022) Bioactive Compounds for Fibromyalgia-like Symptoms: A Narrative Review and Future Perspectives. IJERPH 19:4148. https://doi.org/10.3390/ijerph19074148

24. Abdelrahman KM, Hackshaw KV (2021) Nutritional Supplements for the Treatment of Neuropathic Pain. Biomedicines 9:674. https://doi.org/10.3390/biomedicines9060674

25. Sarzi-Puttini P, Giorgi V, Atzeni F, Gorla R, Kosek E, Choy EH, Bazzichi L, Häuser W, Ablin JN, Aloush V, Buskila D, Amital H, Da Silva JAP, Perrot S, Morlion B, Polati E, Schweiger V, Coaccioli S, Varrassi G, Di Franco M, Torta R, Øien Forseth KM, Mannerkorpi K, Salaffi F, Di Carlo M, Cassisi G, Batticciotto A (2021) Fibromyalgia position paper. Clinical and Experimental Rheumatology 39:186–193. https://doi.org/10.55563/clinexprheumatol/i19pig

26. (2021) Quality of life and psychological assessment in patients with Fibromyalgia Syndrome during COVID-19 pandemic in Italy: prospective observational study. SV. https://doi.org/10.22514/sv.2021.127

27. González-Flores D, López-Pingarrón L, Castaño MY, Gómez MÁ, Rodríguez AB, García JJ, Garrido M (2023) Melatonin as a Coadjuvant in the Treatment of Patients with Fibromyalgia. Biomedicines 11:1964. https://doi.org/10.3390/biomedicines11071964

28. Pallotti F, Bergamini C, Lamperti C, Fato R (2021) The Roles of Coenzyme Q in Disease: Direct and Indirect Involvement in Cellular Functions. IJMS 23:128. https://doi.org/10.3390/ijms23010128

29. Pastor-Maldonado CJ, Suárez-Rivero JM, Povea-Cabello S, Álvarez-Córdoba M, Villalón-García I, Munuera-Cabeza M, Suárez-Carrillo A, Talaverón-Rey M, Sánchez-Alcázar JA (2020) Coenzyme Q10: Novel Formulations and Medical Trends. IJMS 21:8432. https://doi.org/10.3390/ijms21228432

30. Mantle D, Hargreaves IP, Domingo JC, Castro-Marrero J (2024) Mitochondrial Dysfunction and Coenzyme Q10 Supplementation in Post-Viral Fatigue Syndrome: An Overview. IJMS 25:574. https://doi.org/10.3390/ijms25010574

31. Isasi C, Colmenero I, Casco F, Tejerina E, Fernandez N, Serrano-Vela JI, Castro MJ, Villa LF (2014) Fibromyalgia and non-celiac gluten sensitivity: a description with remission of fibromyalgia. Rheumatol Int 34:1607–1612. https://doi.org/10.1007/s00296-014-2990-6

32. Axford JS (1999) Glycosylation and rheumatic disease. Biochimica et Biophysica Acta (BBA) - Molecular Basis of Disease 1455:219–229. https://doi.org/10.1016/S0925-4439(99)00057-5

33. Becker S, Schweinhardt P (2012) Dysfunctional Neurotransmitter Systems in Fibromyalgia, Their Role in Central Stress Circuitry and Pharmacological Actions on These Systems. Pain Research and Treatment 2012:1–10. https://doi.org/10.1155/2012/741746

34. Mehta A, Prabhakar M, Kumar P, Deshmukh R, Sharma PL (2013) Excitotoxicity: Bridge to various triggers in neurodegenerative disorders. European Journal of Pharmacology 698:6–18. https://doi.org/10.1016/j.ejphar.2012.10.032

35. Casini I, Ladisa V, Clemente L, Delussi M, Rostanzo E, Peparini S, Aloisi AM, De Tommaso M (2024) A Personalized Mediterranean Diet Improves Pain and Quality of Life in Patients with Fibromyalgia. Pain Ther 13:609–620. https://doi.org/10.1007/s40122-024-00598-2

36. Castaldo G, Marino C, Atteno M, D'Elia M, Pagano I, Grimaldi M, Conte A, Molettieri P, Santoro A, Napolitano E, Puca I, Raimondo M, Parisella C, D'Ursi AM, Rastrelli L (2024) Investigating the Effectiveness of a Carb-Free Oloproteic Diet in Fibromyalgia Treatment. Nutrients 16:1620. https://doi.org/10.3390/nu16111620

37. Rus A, Molina F, Ramos MM, Martínez-Ramírez MJ, Del Moral ML (2017) Extra Virgin Olive Oil Improves Oxidative Stress, Functional Capacity, and Health-Related Psychological Status in Patients With Fibromyalgia: A Preliminary Study. Biological Research For Nursing 19:106–115. https://doi.org/10.1177/1099800416659370

38. Menzel J, Jabakhanji A, Biemann R, Mai K, Abraham K, Weikert C (2020) Systematic review and meta-analysis of the associations of vegan and vegetarian diets with inflammatory biomarkers. Sci Rep 10:21736. https://doi.org/10.1038/s41598-020-78426-8

39. Nijs J, Elma Ö, Yilmaz ST, Mullie P, Vanderweeën L, Clarys P, Deliens T, Coppieters I, Weltens N, Van Oudenhove L, Malfliet A (2019) Nutritional neurobiology and central nervous system sensitisation: missing link in a comprehensive treatment for chronic pain? British Journal of Anaesthesia 123:539–543. https://doi.org/10.1016/j.bja.2019.07.016

40. Haghighatdoost F, Bellissimo N, Totosy De Zepetnek JO, Rouhani MH (2017) Association of vegetarian diet with inflammatory biomarkers: a systematic review and meta-analysis of observational studies. Public Health Nutr 20:2713–2721. https://doi.org/10.1017/S1368980017001768

41. Fernández-Araque A, Verde Z, Torres-Ortega C, Sainz-Gil M, Velasco-Gonzalez V, González-Bernal JJ, Mielgo-Ayuso J (2022) Effects of Antioxidants on Pain Perception in Patients with Fibromyalgia—A Systematic Review. JCM 11:2462. https://doi.org/10.3390/jcm11092462

42. Carrasco-Querol N, González Serra G, Bueno Hernández N, Gonçalves AQ, Pastor Cazalla M, Bestratén Del Pino P, Montesó Curto P, Caballol Angelats R, Fusté Anguera I, Sancho Sol MC, Castro Blanco E, Vila-Martí A, Medina-Perucha L, Fernández-Sáez J, Dalmau Llorca MR, Aguilar Martín C (2023) Effectiveness and health benefits of a nutritional, chronobiological and physical exercise primary care intervention in fibromyalgia and chronic fatigue syndrome: SYNCHRONIZE + mixed-methods study protocol. Medicine 102:e33637. https://doi.org/10.1097/MD.0000000000033637

43. Bjørklund G, Dadar M, Chirumbolo S, Aaseth J (2018) Fibromyalgia and nutrition: Therapeutic possibilities? Biomedicine & Pharmacotherapy 103:531–538. https://doi.org/10.1016/j.biopha.2018.04.056

Psychological Support and Coping

Clara Nemr

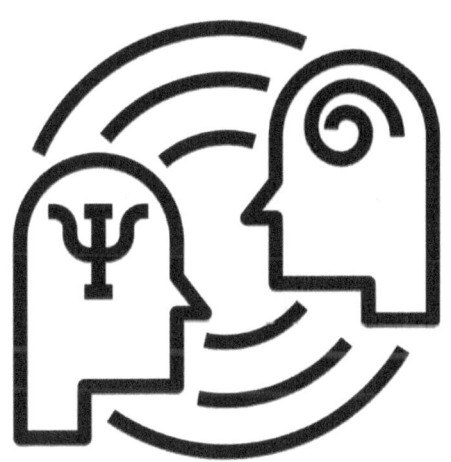

Introduction

Psychological support plays a crucial role in managing fibromyalgia (FM), a chronic condition characterized by widespread pain, fatigue, cognitive difficulties, and other debilitating symptoms. As fibromyalgia significantly impacts both physical and mental well-being, addressing the psychological aspects of the disorder is essential for comprehensive patient care and improved quality of life.

The exact cause of fibromyalgia syndrome (FMS) remains unclear. However, researchers generally agree that changes in both the central and peripheral nervous systems play a significant role. A key area of investigation focuses on identifying the factors that may trigger or predispose individuals to these neurological changes. Such factors could include infections, vaccinations, or physical and psychological trauma. Thus, patients with FM symptoms should receive treatment from a multidisciplinary team, including a psychologist[1].

Psychological aspects of fibromyalgia

Fibromyalgia (FM) is often viewed as a manifestation of emotional distress linked to past traumas or stressful events. These experiences may alter brain function, leading to central sensitization and increased nerve activity. The connection between psychological stress and FM development is supported by the high prevalence of post-traumatic stress disorder (PTSD) and abnormal cortisol levels among FM patients, indicating a significant relationship with chronic pain. Physical factors, such as car accidents and cervical spine injuries, have been identified as potential FM triggers. Some studies suggest a direct link between physical traumas and FM onset, with a higher likelihood of FM following such events[2].

Our understanding of FM has been greatly enhanced by the description of neurophysiological mechanisms like central sensitization, which leads to heightened pain sensitivity. Functional magnetic resonance imaging studies have revealed alterations in pain processing in FM patients, including changes in neurotransmitter levels that suggest disrupted pain modulation. Genetic research has proposed that factors predisposing individuals to FM may include the presence of the Apo E4 allele and altered serum microRNA levels related to pain severity[3].

The relationship between FM and psychological trauma is well-documented, with many patients reporting past traumas often associated with depression. Studies have highlighted a significant link between FM and childhood emotional and sexual abuse, suggesting that psychological traumas can increase the likelihood of developing FM. This connection may be mediated by endocrine factors such as altered cortisol secretion patterns [4].

PTSD and FM share numerous symptoms, including elevated stress levels and reduced quality of life. The high prevalence of PTSD among FM patients and the observation of abnormal cortisol secretion levels due to traumatic events in both disorders support the idea that PTSD and FM are comorbidities with overlapping etiologies. These conditions may emerge in individuals vulnerable to trauma[2].

Determining an individual's likelihood of developing a pathological response to trauma is complex and requires further research in areas such as genetic factors, autonomic sympathetic functioning, and neurotransmitter transmission.

While the literature on the relationship between emotional trauma and FM is extensive, many studies are based on retrospective self-reporting and may be affected by recall bias. Nevertheless, some studies, including those with rheumatological control groups, have found a definite association. Debate continues regarding the type and timing of traumatic events related to FM development, which has been variously associated with childhood abuse, neglect, and adult physical and sexual abuse[5].

The abnormal cortisol secretion observed in FM patients with a history of abuse supports the theory that symptom development may reflect a chronic stress reaction. However, the specificity of this reaction requires further clarification, as it may be influenced by comorbid psychological disorders such as major depressive disorder (MDD), PTSD, and anxiety[4].

The generally poor quality of existing evidence from published studies on the association between FM and psychological trauma highlights the need for more comprehensive research. Future studies should consider both psychological and physical factors to improve the prevention, diagnosis, and treatment of FM.

While physicians frequently observe a connection between trauma and fibromyalgia onset, a comprehensive review of this relationship has been lacking. A literature search identified 31 studies exploring the link between fibromyalgia and prior and psychological trauma. The review found that many studies reported a significant association between psychological trauma and the onset of FM. Several studies indicated that PTSD may play a mediating role in the development of FM following traumatic events. In addition, these studies consistently showed higher rates of psychological trauma in FM patients compared to the general population. The review notes that physicians often encounter patients whose fibromyalgia appears to be precipitated by physical or psychological trauma, highlighting the clinical relevance of this association[4].

Another study investigated the impact of chronic pain and related psychological factors on functional outcomes in FM patients. 91 FM patients completed an online questionnaire assessing pain intensity, pain interference, pain catastrophizing, pain self-efficacy, and health-related quality of life. These findings indicate that psychological factors, particularly catastrophic thinking and self-efficacy, have a more substantial impact on daily functioning, physical well-being, and mental health in FM patients than the intensity of pain itself. These psychological variables appear to be key determinants in shaping the overall health outcomes and quality of life for individuals with FM[6]. These findings show the importance of considering psychological aspects in the etiology and treatment of FM, suggesting that trauma-informed care.

Psychological treatment for fibromyalgia
1. **Cognitive Behavioral Therapy**

The mental health challenges faced by many FM patients can exacerbate physical symptoms and further diminish the quality of life. Thus, psychological treatment can be beneficial in minimizing FM symptoms. Currently, cognitive behavioral therapy (CBT) is the preferred psychological treatment for chronic pain conditions, including FM. CBT focuses on how cognitive interpretations and behaviors influence pain experiences. The therapy is based on the premise that negative beliefs about pain and perceived lack of control can lead to dysfunctional behaviors and emotions, which in turn reinforce pain-related thoughts[7]. Through CBT, patients can identify and modify distorted thoughts about pain, recognize and change dysfunctional behaviors, develop more effective coping strategies, and realize their capacity to manage pain-related challenges[8]. A meta-analysis of 23 randomized controlled trials revealed that CBT significantly reduced pain, sleep disturbances, and depression in FM patients compared to control groups[9]. Another systematic review of 14 studies found that

CBT led to improvements in pain intensity, fatigue, and quality of life, with effects persisting at long-term follow-ups. Additionally, neuroimaging studies have demonstrated that CBT can alter brain activity patterns associated with pain processing in FM patients, suggesting a neurobiological basis for its efficacy[10]. These findings collectively support CBT as a valuable component of comprehensive FM treatment, highlighting its potential to address both psychological and physiological aspects of the condition.

2. Mindfulness-Based Stress Reduction

Mindfulness-Based Stress Reduction (MBSR) has shown promise as a complementary treatment for fibromyalgia, offering potential benefits in managing symptoms and improving the quality of life for patients with this chronic pain condition[11]. A randomized controlled trial evaluated the effects of MBSR on fibromyalgia patients, comparing an MBSR group therapy to a waitlist control group. The study involved 95 fibromyalgia patients and measured outcomes including fibromyalgia symptoms, depression, perceived stress, psychological inflexibility in pain, and pain catastrophizing at pre-intervention, post-intervention, and 6-month follow-up. Overall, the results demonstrated that MBSR led to significant improvements in fibromyalgia symptoms, perceived stress, and depression compared to the control group, with many of these improvements persisting at the 6-month follow-up. Additionally, the study identified psychological inflexibility in pain and pain catastrophizing as important mechanisms of change, suggesting that MBSR's effectiveness is partly due to its ability to modify these pain-related cognitions[12].

3. Sleep Quality

Sleep quality is also important for minimizing FM symptoms. 70 Women with FM received information about the disease and a sleep diary, but only the experimental group was given sleep hygiene instructions. After implementing these practices for three months, all participants were reassessed using initial questionnaires to evaluate the impact of sleep hygiene on their condition. Studies showed that sleep hygiene instructions led to behavioral changes in patients, resulting in reduced pain and fatigue, improved perceived sleep quality, and easier return to sleep after night-time awakenings[13].

4. Acceptance and Commitment Therapy (ACT)

Acceptance and Commitment Therapy (ACT) has shown promising results in helping individuals with fibromyalgia manage their symptoms and improve their quality of life. Several studies have examined the effectiveness of ACT for fibromyalgia: Luciano et al. (2014) conducted a randomized controlled trial with 156 fibromyalgia patients, comparing Group ACT (GACT) to recommended pharmacological treatment (RPT) and a control group. The GACT intervention consisted of eight 2.5-hour sessions covering ACT principles, mindfulness, values, and acceptance strategies. Results showed that GACT was statistically superior to both RPT and the control group immediately after treatment, with improvements maintained at 6 months. GACT improved functional status, pain catastrophizing, and health-related quality of life, with medium effect sizes in most cases[14].

Another study by Wicksell et al. (2013) examined ACT's effectiveness in women with fibromyalgia. The intervention included twelve 90-minute sessions focusing on behavioral changes, shifting perspectives, values-oriented activation, and acceptance strategies. The ACT group showed significant improvements in physical and mental quality of life and reduced fibromyalgia symptoms compared to the control group[15].

A more recent study by Ramos et al. (2024) found that ACT improved mental health, social functioning, and affective problems (such as somatization, obsession-compulsion, depression, and anxiety) in fibromyalgia patients. The improvements were maintained at a six-month follow-up, indicating the long-term effectiveness of ACT[16].

Overall, these studies suggest that ACT is an effective intervention for improving the quality of life and reducing symptoms in individuals with fibromyalgia. ACT appears to be particularly beneficial in enhancing psychological flexibility, pain acceptance, and overall functionality, even when pain levels remain unchanged. The therapy's focus on living a meaningful life despite adverse health conditions aligns well with the management of chronic conditions like fibromyalgia.

5. Hypnosis

Hypnosis has been explored as a potential intervention for improving the quality of life in women with fibromyalgia, though results have been mixed. In a study by Picard et al. (2013), 120 women with fibromyalgia participated in five 1-hour hypnosis sessions conducted by a psychologist. These sessions focused on stress management, breathing techniques, and concentrating on the body and pain. Despite these efforts, the study found no significant improvement in the quality of life or reduction in fibromyalgia symptoms at both 3-month and 6-month follow-ups. The limited number of sessions was suggested as a possible reason for the lack of significant results[17]. However, other studies have shown more promising outcomes. For instance, a study by the National Institute of Health reported that fibromyalgia sufferers using hypnosis experienced an 80% reduction in painful episodes.

Additionally, a randomized controlled trial found that self-administered audio-recorded hypnosis significantly decreased pain intensity, fatigue, and depressive symptoms, suggesting that hypnosis can be a practical and economical alternative for managing fibromyalgia symptoms[18]. These mixed results indicate that while hypnosis has potential benefits, further research with more extensive and varied methodologies is needed to fully understand its efficacy in treating fibromyalgia.

6. Emotional Social Support

Emotional and social support is a key factor in managing fibromyalgia pain symptoms. A study investigated the effects of social support on pain perception and processing in FM patients. Researchers examined pain thresholds, ratings, and brain activity under two conditions: patients alone and with a significant other present. The results showed that FM patients experienced reduced pain sensitivity, lower subjective pain ratings, and decreased brain activity at tender points when their significant other was present, compared to being alone. These effects were not observed in migraine patients, suggesting that social support may uniquely influence pain processing in FM at other behavioral and neurological levels[19].

7. Meditation

Mindfulness meditation has shown promise as a complementary approach for managing fibromyalgia symptoms. A comprehensive review of seven experimental studies on mindfulness interventions for fibromyalgia patients revealed several positive outcomes. Most interventions consisted of multiple group sessions spanning several months. While the effectiveness varied across studies, the most consistent improvements were observed in anxiety, depression, sleep-related symptoms, coping abilities, and perceived stress levels[20]. These benefits may be attributed to increases in self-compassion and psychological flexibility fostered by mindfulness practices. For instance, a study demonstrated significant improvements (40-50%) in fibromyalgia symptoms through mindfulness meditation[21]. Another randomized clinical trial found that meditation significantly reduced perceived stress, sleep disturbance, and symptom severity in fibromyalgia patients, with benefits maintained at a two-month follow-up[22]. While the evidence is not yet sufficient to recommend mindfulness as a comprehensive management strategy for all fibromyalgia symptoms, it shows promise in addressing mood- and sleep-related issues. Researchers suggest that further rigorous studies are needed to fully establish the efficacy of mindfulness interventions for fibromyalgia.

8. Music Therapy

A study by Weber et al. (2015) investigated the effects of music therapy, vibration, and their combination on women with fibromyalgia. The research involved 120 women randomly divided into four groups: Music Therapy, Vibration, Complete (music + vibration), and Control. Participants underwent five 30-minute sessions over several days, with vibration transducers placed on specific acupuncture points. The study found that music therapy improved the quality of life in women with fibromyalgia, with all intervention groups showing significant improvements in the Fibromyalgia Impact Questionnaire (FIQ) and Health Assessment Questionnaire (HAQ) scores. Notably, the Complete group exhibited the best results, suggesting a potential synergistic effect of combining music therapy with vibration[23]. These findings highlight the promise of non-pharmacological interventions in managing fibromyalgia symptoms. However, the study had limitations, including a short intervention period and lack of long-term follow-up.

Further research is needed to explore the long-term effects, optimal intervention durations, and mechanisms behind the observed improvements. Despite these limitations, this study provides valuable evidence for the potential use of music therapy and vibration in improving the quality of life and symptoms of women with fibromyalgia, paving the way for more comprehensive investigations in this area[23].

9. Dance

Research has shown that dance, a physical activity with psychosocial benefits, may positively impact pain management in FM patients. A systematic review aimed to investigate the effect of dance interventions on pain through quantitative measures and qualitative themes. Seven major databases were searched from inception to January 2021, and studies were included if the dance interventions lasted more than 6 weeks, participants reported pain for longer than 3 months, and pain was an outcome. Out of 23,628 articles, 34 full papers were included, involving 1,254 participants, predominantly female. The studies mainly focused on individuals with fibromyalgia (26%) and generalized chronic pain (14%), with aerobic dance and Biodanza being the most common genres. Results showed that 74% of studies noted reduced pain through quantitative measures or qualitative themes of improved pain experience, with 88% improvement for chronic primary pain and 80% for chronic secondary musculoskeletal pain. The review concluded that dance interventions, particularly those lasting 60-150 minutes weekly, had positive effects on chronic pain, suggesting dance is an effective adjunct in chronic pain management [24].

10. Climate and seasonal variations

Climatic and seasonal factors, particularly changes in barometric pressure and temperature, have been shown to significantly impact the symptoms of fibromyalgia (FM). Research indicates that fluctuations in barometric pressure, especially those preceding storms, can exacerbate pain in FM patients. A study involving 48 participants found that low barometric pressure combined with high humidity levels led to increased pain and stress, with notable individual variations in response[25]. Temperature also plays a role in FM symptom management. Cold weather tends to increase stiffness and pain, while heat can worsen fatigue. Some researchers have proposed a link between anomalies in temperature perception among FM patients and the connection between thermoregulatory dysfunctions and pain.

The relationship between seasonal changes and FM symptoms has been explored in connection with seasonal affective disorder (SAD). However, research findings in this area are mixed. One study involving 471 FM patients found no significant seasonal impact on symptoms. In contrast, another study with 1,424 patients suffering from various rheumatic diseases, including FM, observed seasonal variations in reported symptom severity[26]. Interestingly, these self-reported fluctuations were not corroborated by clinical measurements, suggesting a potential discrepancy between patients' perceptions and objective clinical assessments. These findings highlight the complex interplay between environmental factors and FM symptoms, emphasizing the need for individualized approaches to symptom management and further research to better understand these relationships.

Research indicates that FM patients display diverse psychological profiles. Thus, personalized treatment approaches are crucial for effective management of FMS. These interventions should address patient needs, respond to patient progress, and utilize measurement-based care with regular outcome monitoring[11].

Conclusion

In conclusion, this chapter highlights the critical role of psychological support and coping strategies in the management of fibromyalgia. The complex interplay between psychological factors and physical symptoms in FM necessitates a multidisciplinary approach to treatment.

Cognitive behavioral therapy, mindfulness-based stress reduction, sleep hygiene interventions, and social support have all demonstrated efficacy in improving various aspects of FM, from pain perception to overall quality of life. These findings show the importance of addressing psychological trauma, catastrophic thinking, and self-efficacy in FM patients. Moreover, the research suggests that personalized, trauma-informed care that considers individual psychological profiles can lead to better outcomes. Moving forward, healthcare providers should consider integrating these psychological approaches into comprehensive FM treatment plans. Future research should focus on refining these interventions, exploring their long-term effects, and investigating potential synergies between psychological and pharmacological treatments. By continuing to enhance our understanding of the psychological aspects of FM, we can develop more effective, patient-centered strategies to improve the lives of those living with this challenging condition.

References:

1. Luciano JV, Neblett R, Peñacoba C, Suso-Ribera C, McCracken LM (2023) The Contribution of the Psychologist in the Assessment and Treatment of Fibromyalgia. Curr Treat Options in Rheum 9:11–31. https://doi.org/10.1007/s40674-023-00200-4

2. Redelmeier DA, Zung JD, Thiruchelvam D, Tibshirani RJ (2015) Fibromyalgia and the Risk of a Subsequent Motor Vehicle Crash. J Rheumatol 42:1502–1510. https://doi.org/10.3899/jrheum.141315

3. Bjersing JL, Bokarewa MI, Mannerkorpi K (2015) Profile of circulating microRNAs in fibromyalgia and their relation to symptom severity: an exploratory study. Rheumatol Int 35:635–642. https://doi.org/10.1007/s00296-014-3139-3

4. Yavne Y, Amital D, Watad A, Tiosano S, Amital H (2018) A systematic review of precipitating physical and psychological traumatic events in the development of fibromyalgia. Seminars in Arthritis and Rheumatism 48:121–133. https://doi.org/10.1016/j.semarthrit.2017.12.011

5. Alciati A, Cirillo M, Masala IF, Sarzi-Puttini P, Atzeni F (2021) Differences in depression, anxiety and stress disorders between fibromyalgia associated with rheumatoid arthritis and primary fibromyalgia. Stress and Health 37:255–262. https://doi.org/10.1002/smi.2992

6. Mellace D, Aiello EN, Del Prete-Ferrucci G, De Sandi A, Marfoli A, Ruggiero F, Mameli F, Prandin R, Curti B, De Luca G, Chieffo D, Poletti B, Pravettoni G, Priori A, Barbieri S, Ferrucci R (2024) Beyond pain: the influence of psychological factors on functional status in fibromyalgia. Clinical and Experimental Rheumatology. https://doi.org/10.55563/clinexprheumatol/9qrqel
7. Skinner M, Wilson HD, Turk DC (2012) Cognitive-Behavioral Perspective and Cognitive-Behavioral Therapy for People With Chronic Pain: Distinctions, Outcomes, and Innovations. J Cogn Psychother 26:93–113. https://doi.org/10.1891/0889-8391.26.2.93
8. Gatchel RJ, Peng YB, Peters ML, Fuchs PN, Turk DC (2007) The biopsychosocial approach to chronic pain: Scientific advances and future directions. Psychological Bulletin 133:581–624. https://doi.org/10.1037/0033-2909.133.4.581
9. Thieme K, Mathys M, Turk DC (2017) Evidenced-Based Guidelines on the Treatment of Fibromyalgia Patients: Are They Consistent and If Not, Why Not? Have Effective Psychological Treatments Been Overlooked? The Journal of Pain 18:747–756. https://doi.org/10.1016/j.jpain.2016.12.006
10. Alda M, Luciano JV, Andrés E, Serrano-Blanco A, Rodero B, Del Hoyo Y, Roca M, Moreno S, Magallón R, García-Campayo J (2011) Effectiveness of cognitive behaviour therapy for the treatment of catastrophisation in patients with fibromyalgia: a randomised controlled trial. Arthritis Res Ther 13:R173. https://doi.org/10.1186/ar3496

11. Gual-Montolio P, Martínez-Borba V, Bretón-López JM, Osma J, Suso-Ribera C (2020) How Are Information and Communication Technologies Supporting Routine Outcome Monitoring and Measurement-Based Care in Psychotherapy? A Systematic Review. IJERPH 17:3170. https://doi.org/10.3390/ijerph17093170

12. Taub R, Agmon-Levin N, Frumer L, Samuel-Magal I, Glick I, Horesh D (2024) Mindfulness-based stress reduction (MBSR) for fibromyalgia patients: The role of pain cognitions as mechanisms of change. Complementary Therapies in Clinical Practice 56:101860. https://doi.org/10.1016/j.ctcp.2024.101860

13. Orlandi AC, Ventura C, Gallinaro AL, Costa RA, Lage LV (2012) Improvement in pain, fatigue, and subjective sleep quality through sleep hygiene tips in patients with fibromyalgia. Rev Bras Reumatol 52:666–678

14. Luciano JV, Guallar JA, Aguado J, López-del-Hoyo Y, Olivan B, Magallón R, Alda M, Serrano-Blanco A, Gili M, Garcia-Campayo J (2014) Effectiveness of group acceptance and commitment therapy for fibromyalgia: A 6-month randomized controlled trial (EFFIGACT study). Pain 155:693–702. https://doi.org/10.1016/j.pain.2013.12.029

15. Wicksell RK, Kemani M, Jensen K, Kosek E, Kadetoff D, Sorjonen K, Ingvar M, Olsson GL (2013) Acceptance and commitment therapy for fibromyalgia: A randomized controlled trial. European Journal of Pain 17:599–611. https://doi.org/10.1002/j.1532-2149.2012.00224.x

16. Ramos C, Ríos FL, Muñante GP, Ordóñez-Carrasco J (2024) Group Acceptance and Commitment Therapy (ACT) for Fibromyalgia Patients. Clínica y Salud 35:39–48. https://doi.org/10.5093/clysa2024a1
17. Picard P, Jusseaume C, Boutet M, Dualé C, Mulliez A, Aublet-Cuvellier B (2013) Hypnosis for Management of Fibromyalgia. International Journal of Clinical and Experimental Hypnosis 61:111–123. https://doi.org/10.1080/00207144.2013.729441
18. Fisch S, Brinkhaus B, Teut M (2017) Hypnosis in patients with perceived stress - a systematic review. BMC Complement Altern Med 17:323. https://doi.org/10.1186/s12906-017-1806-0
19. Montoya P, Larbig W, Braun C, Preissl H, Birbaumer N (2004) Influence of social support and emotional context on pain processing and magnetic brain responses in fibromyalgia. Arthritis & Rheumatism 50:4035–4044. https://doi.org/10.1002/art.20660
20. Gordon S, Brown R, Hogan M, Menzies V (2023) Mindfulness as a Symptom Management Strategy for Fibromyalgia: An Integrative Review. J Holist Nurs 41:200–214. https://doi.org/10.1177/08980101221123833
21. Kaplan KH, Goldenberg DL, Galvin-Nadeau M (1993) The impact of a meditation-based stress reduction program on fibromyalgia. General Hospital Psychiatry 15:284–289. https://doi.org/10.1016/0163-8343(93)90020-O

22. Cash E, Salmon P, Weissbecker I, Rebholz WN, Bayley-Veloso R, Zimmaro LA, Floyd A, Dedert E, Sephton SE (2015) Mindfulness meditation alleviates fibromyalgia symptoms in women: results of a randomized clinical trial. Ann Behav Med 49:319–330. https://doi.org/10.1007/s12160-014-9665-0

23. Weber A, Werneck L, Paiva E, Gans P (2015) Effects of Music in Combination with Vibration in Acupuncture Points on the Treatment of Fibromyalgia. The Journal of Alternative and Complementary Medicine 21:77–82. https://doi.org/10.1089/acm.2014.0199

24. Hickman B, Pourkazemi F, Pebdani RN, Hiller CE, Fong Yan A (2022) Dance for Chronic Pain Conditions: A Systematic Review. Pain Medicine 23:2022–2041. https://doi.org/10.1093/pm/pnac092

25. Fagerlund AJ, Iversen M, Ekeland A, Moen CM, Aslaksen PM (2019) Blame it on the weather? The association between pain in fibromyalgia, relative humidity, temperature and barometric pressure. PLoS ONE 14:e0216902. https://doi.org/10.1371/journal.pone.0216902

26. Castel A, Poveda MJ, Rodríguez-Muguruza S, Castro S, Fontova R (2023) Relación entre la estación del año y la gravedad de los síntomas en pacientes con fibromialgia. Medicina Clínica 160:60–65. https://doi.org/10.1016/j.medcli.2022.04.009

Medication management for fibromyalgia

Philo Antoun

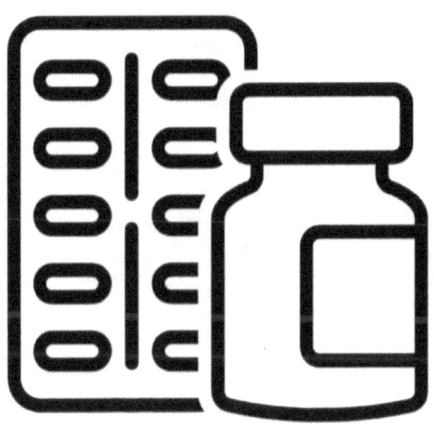

Transition

While psychological support and coping mechanisms play an important role in treating fibromyalgia, they can be complemented with pharmacological medication to achieve the best results. Psychological interventions, like cognitive-behavioral therapy (CBT), help patients manage the emotional and mental aspects of pain associated with fibromyalgia by decreasing stress and anxiety[1]. However, many patients are still left with physical pain, fatigue, and disturbed sleep cycles. As a result, an integrated strategy with psychological and pharmacological approaches is the best for managing this multifaceted illness[1]. The following sections will focus on specific classes of medications used in fibromyalgia, their mechanisms of action, pharmacodynamics, contraindications, side effects, and dosing guidelines, providing a comprehensive overview of medication management in fibromyalgia.

The Significance of Medication Management in Patients with Fibromyalgia

Medication management plays an important role in fibromyalgia treatment because of the complex nature of the illness. As discussed, this illness can affect the body in a variety of ways, thereby underscoring the importance of developing a patient-centered approach when deciding on a treatment plan.

Medications Used in Fibromyalgia

Antidepressants

Tricyclic Antidepressants (TCAs)

Mechanism of Action

Tricyclic Antidepressants (TCAs) work by inhibiting the presynaptic reuptake of serotonin and norepinephrine, resulting in an increase in their levels in the central nervous system. This mechanism is useful in alleviating neuropathic pain, and TCAs impact descending pain pathways by strengthening the body's ability to inhibit pain signals[2-7].

Names of Medications in this class

Amitriptyline

Pharmacodynamics and Pharmacokinetics

TCAs are used to treat patients who have major depression, OCD, nocturnal enuresis, peripheral neuropathy, and sleep abnormalities, which is relevant for patients who have fibromyalgia. When administered orally, TCAs undergo first-pass metabolism in the liver. They are well absorbed with a bioavailability of 40-50%, have a long half-life of about 10-50 hours, and are a substrate of the CYP2D6 system[2-6].

Side Effects/Contraindications/Dosing

These medications are contraindicated in patients with a recent or a history of myocardial infarction, heart block, and those taking MAOI inhibitors. Common side effects include dry mouth, urinary retention, tachycardia, and confusion. Other serious side effects can include cardiac arrhythmias leading to Torsades de pointes and orthostatic hypotension. When starting patients on TCAs, they can begin on a low dose of 10-25 mg and tailor the dosage based on their response and tolerance[2-7].

Serotonin-norepinephrine reuptake Inhibitors (SNRIs)

Mechanism of Action

SNRIs increase the levels of serotonin (5-HT) and norepinephrine (NE) in the brain by inhibiting the reuptake mechanisms of both neurotransmitters, serotonin transporter (SERT) and norepinephrine transporter (NET)[2-8].

Names of Medications in this class

Duloxetine, Milnacipran, Venlafaxine, Reboxetine, and Esreboxetine

Pharmacodynamics and Pharmacokinetics

Duloxetine and milnacipran are well absorbed orally and approved for fibromyalgia in adolescents 13 years and older. Both drugs are used in patients with peripheral neuropathy. Duloxetine has a bioavailability of 50% and is metabolized by CYP1A2 and CYP2D6, while milnacipran has a bioavailability of 85% and is not metabolized as much but rather excreted in urine[2-8].

Side Effects/Contraindications/Dosing

SNRIs are contraindicated in patients with hypertension and any history of liver disease. Side effects include sedation, nausea, sympathetic activation, and increased blood pressure. Duloxetine is usually started at 30 mg daily and increased to 60 mg daily, while milnacipran is started at 12.5 mg daily and increased to 50 mg twice daily[2,3].

Selective Serotonin Reuptake Inhibitors (SSRIs)

Mechanism of Action

SSRIs work by blocking the reabsorption of serotonin and allosterically inhibiting the serotonin transporter (SERT), thereby increasing Serotonin in the synapse, which helps with mood, pain, and anxiety[2,4,5,6].

Names of Medications in this class

Fluoxetine, Citalopram, Escitalopram, and Paroxetine

Pharmacodynamics and Pharmacokinetics

SSRIs help with depressive disorders, generalized anxiety disorder, PTSD, panic disorder, OCD, bulimia, premenstrual dysphoric disorder, and premature ejaculation. Fluoxetine is a CYP2D6 inhibitor with a high bioavailability of 70% and long half of 48-72 hours[2,4,5,6].

Side Effects/Contraindications/Dosing

SSRIs are contraindicated in patients taking MAOI inhibitors and should be used with caution with those with bipolar disorder because they can induce mania. Side effects may include serotonin syndrome, sexual dysfunction, nausea, vomiting, and weight gain. Fluoxetine can be started at 20 mg daily and tailored to patient response[2,4-6].

Anticonvulsants

Gabapentinoids

Mechanism of Action

Gabapentinoids bind to the alpha-2-delta subunit of voltage-gated calcium channels in the central nervous system and inhibit the release of excitatory neurotransmitters[2,4-7].

Names of Medications in this class

Gabapentin, Pregabalin, Lacosamide, and Carbamazepine

Pharmacodynamics and Pharmacokinetics

Gabapentinoids reduce pain and improve sleep. They are used for neuropathic pain and prevent partial seizures. It is important to highlight that although gabapentin is a GABA analog, it does not bind or affect the GABA receptors. Gabapentin and pregabalin are well absorbed orally, have half-lives of around six hours, and are metabolized in the gastrointestinal tract. Finally, the bioavailability of Gabapentin decreases as the dose is increased[2,4-7].

Side Effects/Contraindications/Dosing

Gabapentinoids are contraindicated in pregnant patients and or any history of kidney disease. Common side effects include headache, nausea and vomiting, fever, memory loss, and weight gain. Gabapentin can be started at 100-300 mg at bedtime and can be increased up to 1800-2400 mg daily. Pregabalin begins at around 75 mg twice daily and can be increased to 150 mg twice daily[2,4-7].

Muscle Relaxants

Mechanism of Action

Cyclobenzaprine primarily works at the brain stem and is a 5-HT2 receptor antagonist that inhibits the CNS's muscle spasm reflex[5,6,9,10].

Names of Medications in this class

Cyclobenzaprine

Pharmacodynamics and Pharmacokinetics

This medication has been shown to improve the range of motion in MSK conditions, reduce local tenderness, and help with sleep disturbances in fibromyalgia patients. Cyclobenzaprine has a long half-life of about 18 hours and is metabolized by cytochrome P450 enzymes

(CYP3A4, CYP31A2, and CYP2D6) in the liver. It has a bioavailability of about 55% and is excreted by the kidneys and urine[5,6,9,10].

Side Effects/Contraindications/Dosing

It is usually prescribed at 5-10 mg daily and can be increased depending on tolerance. Some side effects include nausea, tachycardia, dizziness, diarrhea, and serotonin syndrome. This medication is contraindicated in patients with heart failure, hyperthyroidism, arrhythmias, or taking any MAOIs[5,6,9,10].

Benzodiazepines

Mechanism of Action

Clonazepam is a long-acting benzodiazepine that binds to the GABA-A receptor, which increases Cl channel frequency and results in decreased neuronal firing via hyperpolarization in the cell[2].

Names of Medications in this class

Clonazepam

Pharmacodynamics and Pharmacokinetics

Benzodiazepines are used in fibromyalgia for its anxiolytic and muscle relaxant effects. Clonazepam helps with insomnia, muscle pain, and panic disorders. It is well absorbed orally with a bioavailability of around 90%. Clonazepam has a half-life of 30-40 hours, metabolized primarily in the liver, and is mainly excreted in the urine[2].

Side Effects/Contraindications/Dosing

Patients start on 0.25-0.5 mg at bedtime, and physicians can increase dosages based on response. Some side effects include nausea, dizziness, diarrhea, and confusion. This medication is contraindicated in patients with a history of substance abuse and should be used with caution in patients with severe respiratory depression[2].

Sleep Aids/Sedatives

Mechanism of Action

Zolpidem and Escopiclone are sedative-hypnotics that act on GABA (BZ1) receptors. However, these medications have a lower risk of dependence than benzodiazepines[2,11].

Names of Medications in this class

Zolpidem and Eszopiclone

Pharmacodynamics and Pharmacokinetics

Non-benzodiazepine hypnotics are utilized to improve the quality of sleep in fibromyalgia patients. Zolpidem has a half-life of 2-3 hours and is metabolized in the gastrointestinal tract by cytochrome P450 enzymes in the liver before being renally excreted. Eszopiclone is metabolized by CYP3A, has a half-life of 6 hours, and is excreted in the urine[2,11].

Side Effects/Contraindications/Dosing

Zolpidem is prescribed at 5-10 mg daily, while eszopiclone is started at 1-3 mg. When using these medications, some side effects may include nausea, headache, and irregular sleep behaviors. Some contraindications include older patient populations who have liver or respiratory disease[2,11].

Antipsychotics

Mechanism of Action

Quetiapine is an atypical antipsychotic agent that can help with sleep disturbances. It's an antagonist at 5-HT2A receptors for serotonin and D1 and D2 receptors for dopamine[2].

Names of Medications in this class

Quetiapine

Pharmacodynamics and Pharmacokinetics

Quetiapine is used to aid with sleep, and it's a mood modulator in patients with mood disorders. This drug can cause suicidal ideation and should not be given to children under 10 years old. Quetiapine is well absorbed orally, metabolized by cytochrome P450 enzymes in the liver, and excreted in the urine. The average half-life of quetiapine is around 6-7 hours [2].

Side Effects/Contraindications/Dosing

With regards to dosage, patients start low at 25 mg at bedtime and can increase depending on response and tolerance. Common side effects include dizziness, weight gain, headache, and constipation. Finally, quetiapine is contraindicated in patients with an arrhythmia, hypotension, history of stroke, or neuroleptic malignant syndrome[2].

Beta-Blockers

Mechanism of Action

Propranolol is a competitive, non-selective beta-blocker that aids in improving sleep quality in fibromyalgia patients and works by blocking hormones such as adrenaline, slowing down the heart rate. When these receptors are blocked, it results in vasoconstriction and inhibition of endothelial growth factor and downregulation of the renin-angiotensin system[2].

Names of Medications in this class

Propranolol

Pharmacodynamics and Pharmacokinetics

Beta Blockers are used in fibromyalgia patients for its anxiolytic and autonomic stabilizing effects. Propranolol is metabolized in the liver by cytochrome p450 enzymes, has a half-life of 3-6 hours, and is excreted in the urine. Finally, propranolol has a bioavailability of about 25%[2].

Side Effects/Contraindications/Dosing

This medication is given at a low dose of 10-20 mg twice daily, which can be increased depending on tolerance. Some side effects include nausea, hypotension, sleeplessness, and fatigue. It is contraindicated in pregnant patients, patients with asthma, and patients with heart failure[2].

Analgesics/Over-the-counter Medications

Mechanism of Action

Both medications block the synthesis of prostaglandins from arachidonic acid via the enzymes COX-1 and COX-2. However, the difference is that acetaminophen only works in the CNS, while NSAIDs work in the brain and throughout the rest of the body. These mechanisms increase the pain threshold[2,11].

Names of Medications in this class

Acetaminophen and NSAIDs

Pharmacodynamics and Pharmacokinetics

Acetaminophen and NSAIDs are, at times, used for pain and symptomatic relief in fibromyalgia. However, their effectiveness is limited compared to the other medications discussed. Both are well absorbed orally, rapidly metabolized in the liver, and have a half-life of about 2-4 hours[2,6,11].

Side Effects/Contraindications/Dosing

Common side effects include increased liver enzymes, stomach pain, heartburn, nausea, and vomiting. Dosing for ibuprofen is 200-400 mg every 4-6 hours as needed, and for acetaminophen, it's 500-1000 mg every 4-6 hours as needed[2,11].

Opioids

Mechanism of Action

Tramadol, a synthetic opioid, binds to μ receptors that inhibit serotonin and norepinephrine reuptake, resulting in decreased pain[5-7,12,13].

Names of Medications in this class

Tramadol

Pharmacodynamics and Pharmacokinetics

Tramadol is an opioid synthetic analgesic that is used in some specific cases of fibromyalgia when pain is severe. Its bioavailability is around 90%, metabolized by cytochrome p450 enzymes in the liver, and has a half-life of around six hours. The kidneys excrete Tramadol[5-7,12,13].

Side Effects/Contraindications/Dosing

Tramadol can be started at 25-50 mg every 4-6 hours and has a maximum dose of 400 mg per day. Common side effects include nausea, drowsiness, constipation, sweating, and risk of dependence. Tramadol is contraindicated in patients with a history of substance abuse, head injury, and severe respiratory depression[5-7,12,13].

Topical Agents

Mechanism of Action

Lidocaine patches reduce pain via local anesthesia by blocking sodium channels. Capsaicin cream functions by decreasing substance P, which is a natural neurotransmitter in our bodies that is involved in pain signaling[12].

Names of Medications in this class

Lidocaine patches and Capsaicin Cream

Pharmacodynamics and Pharmacokinetics

Lidocaine patches and Capsaicin cream are topical medications that provide pain relief in patients with fibromyalgia. These topical agents are well absorbed through the skin and aim to help with neuropathic pain by decreasing the epidermal nerve fibers[12].

Side Effects/Contraindications/Dosing

Lidocaine patches can be applied for up to 12 hours during 24 hours. Side effects include mild skin irritation. Capsaicin cream can be applied multiple times daily and has only mild side effects, including a burning sensation and local irritation. The only contraindication to these topical agents is if the patient has a known sensitivity to these treatments[12].

Experimental Medications

IMC-1

Mechanism of Action

IMC-1 is a combination drug of famciclovir and celecoxib that has the potential to reduce pain and fatigue in fibromyalgia. IMC-1 targets HSV tissue cells by interfering with viral reactivation and lytic infection, which researchers have speculated may trigger fibromyalgia symptoms[5,12].

Names of Medications in this class

IMC-1

Pharmacodynamics and Pharmacokinetics

The absorption and metabolism of IMC-1 consists of the

breakdown of famciclovir and celecoxib. Famciclovir inhibits DNA polymerase, while celecoxib is broken down by cytochrome p450 enzymes[5,12].

Side Effects/Contraindications/Dosing

Because IMC-1 is still under experimental trials, dosing cannot be determined, but this drug is contraindicated in patients with hypersensitivity to famciclovir or celecoxib. However, side effects that patients may experience when using this drug are gastrointestinal side effects like diarrhea, cramps, stomach pain, and vomiting.

Flupirtine

Mechanism of Action

Flupirtine is a non-opioid analgesic that can be used in some cases for its muscle-relaxant properties. It's an NMDA antagonist that activates potassium channels, resulting in pain relief in fibromyalgia patients[5,12].

Names of Medications in this class

Flupirtine

Pharmacodynamics and Pharmacokinetics

Flupirtine has a bioavailability of 90%, is metabolized by the liver, is well absorbed orally, and excreted by the urine. It has an average half-life of around 6.5 hours[5,12].

Side Effects/Contraindications/Dosing

Although Flupirtine may have promising effects, it's not used as often because of its hepatotoxicity, drowsiness, and limited availability. This drug is contraindicated in patients with a previous history of liver or renal disease. With regards to dosing, Flupirtine is still being investigated[5,12].

Ketamine

Mechanism of Action

Ketamine is a general anesthetic that blocks NMDA receptors and can be used as a muscle relaxant to reduce muscle pain in fibromyalgia patients[5].

Names of Medications in this class

Ketamine

Pharmacodynamics and Pharmacokinetics

Ketamine is well absorbed rapidly because it is given intravenously. It has a bioavailability of around 93% and undergoes hepatic metabolism. Ketamine has a half-life of 2-3 hours and is broken down by cytochrome p450 enzymes. It is primarily excreted in the urine[5].

Side Effects/Contraindications/Dosing

Ketamine is still being researched for the most optimal dosing and protocols for fibromyalgia. Side effects include hallucinations, nausea, and dissociation. It is contraindicated in patients with schizophrenia and hypertension[5].

Sodium Oxybate

Mechanism of Action

Sodium oxybate is a CNS depressant that works by breaking down GABA and increasing slow-wave and REM sleep[5,11].

Names of Medications in this class

Sodium Oxybate

Pharmacodynamics and Pharmacokinetics

Sodium oxybate has been researched to reduce pain fatigue, and improve sleep in patients with fibromyalgia. It is rapidly absorbed and metabolized into carbon dioxide and water and has a half-life of 30-60 minutes[5,11].

Side Effects/Contraindications/Dosing

Because it has a high risk for abuse, this medication is still in the experimental stage for fibromyalgia, and dosing cannot be determined. Some side effects include nausea, confusion, and dizziness. It is contraindicated in patients with respiratory disorders[5,6].

Cannabis

Mechanism of Action

Cannabinoids stimulate CB1 and CB2 receptors within the endocannabinoid system, which helps with pain modulation and mood[2,5-7,14].

Names of Medications in this class

Cannabis- THC & CBD

Pharmacodynamics and Pharmacokinetics

Cannabis has been researched for its analgesic and anti-inflammatory effects in fibromyalgia. THC is rapidly absorbed when inhaled, and it is metabolized by the liver by cytochrome p450 enzymes. THC has a half-life of approximately 20-30 hours and is excreted through the feces[5-7,14].

Side Effects/Contraindications/Dosing

More clinical trials are needed to establish efficacy and safety guidelines when treating fibromyalgia patients. Side effects include nausea, drowsiness, dry mouth, and risk for dependence. Cannabis is contraindicated in patients with psychotic disorders and a history of cardiovascular illness[5].

Summary/Transition

Overall, the pharmacological management of fibromyalgia includes a variety of medications that target different symptoms that may arise from fibromyalgia. From antidepressants and anticonvulsants to muscle relaxants and experimental therapies, these medications focus on reducing pain, promoting better sleep, and enhancing the quality of life for fibromyalgia patients. Treatment plans must be individualized and tailored to each patient's symptoms and previous treatment responses.

In the next chapter, we will focus on the role of interventional pain management, and it is important to highlight the clinical implications of these pharmacological strategies. Future research should continue to investigate and optimize existing treatments and develop comprehensive approaches to manage fibromyalgia effectively.

References:

1. "Fibromyalgia." National Institute of Arthritis and Musculoskeletal and Skin Diseases, U.S. Department of Health and Human Services, 23 July 2024, www.niams.nih.gov/health-topics/fibromyalgia/diagnosis-treatment-and-steps-to-take.
2. Buttner, Robert. "Top 200 Drugs Archives." Life in the Fast Lane • LITFL, 26 Feb. 2021, litfl.com/category/basic-science/pharmacology/top-200-drugs/.
3. Chad S Boomershine, MD. "Fibromyalgia Medication." Analgesics, Antianxiety Agents, Skeletal Muscle Relaxants, Antidepressants, Anticonvulsants, Alpha2 Agonists, Medscape, 27 Mar. 2024, emedicine.medscape.com/article/329838-medication#6.
4. Moret, Chantal, and Mike Briley. "Antidepressants in the Treatment of Fibromyalgia." Neuropsychiatric Disease and Treatment, U.S. National Library of Medicine, Dec. 2006, www.ncbi.nlm.nih.gov/pmc/articles/PMC2671948/.
5. Liao, Sharon. "Fibromyalgia: Treatment and Medications." WebMD, WebMD, 2024, www.webmd.com/fibromyalgia/medicines-to-treat-fibromyalgia.
6. Northcott, Melissa J, et al. "Pharmacological Treatment Options for Fibromyalgia." The Pharmaceutical Journal, 12 Feb. 2021, pharmaceutical-journal.com/article/research/pharmacological-treatment-options-for-fibromyalgia.

7. Jurado-Priego, Lina Noelia, et al. "Fibromyalgia: A Review of the Pathophysiological Mechanisms and Multidisciplinary Treatment Strategies." Biomedicines vol. 12,7 1543. 11 Jul. 2024, doi:10.3390/biomedicines12071543

8. "Serotonin Norepinephrine Reuptake Inhibitors (SNRIs)." Elsevier's Healthcare Hub, Elsevier. Health/en-US/preview/serotonin-norepinephrine-reuptake-inhibitors-snris. Accessed 30 July 2024.

9. "DrugBank Online: Database for Drug and Drug Target Info." DrugBank Online | Database for Drug and Drug Target Info, go.drugbank.com/. Accessed 31 July 2024.

10. Tzadok, Roie, and Jacob N Ablin. "Current and Emerging Pharmacotherapy for Fibromyalgia." Pain research & management vol. 2020 6541798. 11 Feb. 2020, doi:10.1155/2020/6541798

11. Mease, Philip J et al. "Pharmacotherapy of fibromyalgia." Best practice & research. Clinical rheumatology vol. 25,2 (2011): 285-97. doi: 10.1016/j.berh.2011.01.015

12. Lawson, Kim. "Emerging Pharmacological Strategies for the Treatment of Fibromyalgia." World Journal of Pharmacology, Baishideng Publishing Group Inc., 9 Mar. 2017, www.wjgnet.com/2220-3192/full/v6/i1/1.htm.

13. Ngian, Gene-Siew, et al. "The use of opioids in fibromyalgia." International journal of rheumatic diseases vol. 14,1 (2011): 6-11. doi:10.1111/j.1756-185X.2010.01567.x

14. Bourke, Stephanie L et al. "Cannabinoids and the endocannabinoid system in fibromyalgia: A review of preclinical and clinical research." Pharmacology & therapeutics vol. 240 (2022): 108216. doi: 10.1016/j.pharmthera.2022.108216

Role of interventional pain

Milan Patel

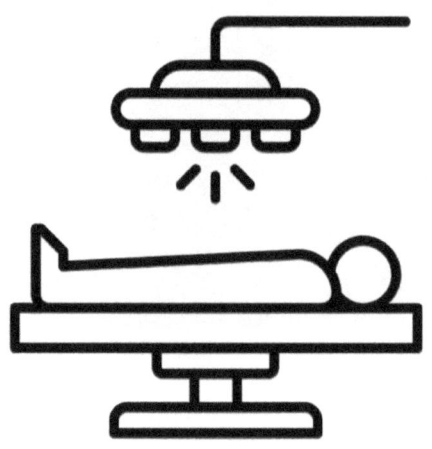

Fibromyalgia indications for interventional pain

Fibromyalgia pain is classified as chronic pain and can be in the realm of interventional pain management. Indications can include but are not limited to widespread musculoskeletal pain, stiffness, and muscle weakness[1]. The prevalence of fibromyalgia is about 2-4% of the population, with women being affected at greater rates.

The central nervous system is the area of the brain that processes pain signals. In fibromyalgic individuals, these pain signals are amplified and sent throughout the body[1]. There is a suspected neurogenic origin, although not entirely certain, with a malfunction of the central nervous system causing hypersensitivity to pain among individuals diagnosed with fibromyalgia[2].

How can interventional pain help

As previously mentioned, fibromyalgia differs from other acute injuries because it falls into the category of chronic pain. Fibromyalgia is aching pain that can last for what seems like a lifetime. However, with interventional pain management, a long-term solution could be closer than one might believe.

Interventional pain management can help with managing the symptoms associated with fibromyalgia. This begins with targeting the source of the pain signals coming from the brain, which can be handled through various interventional pain procedures. Many procedures in the next chapter will go into depth on how neuromodulation can help with reducing and alleviating pain symptoms, specifically with fibromyalgia patients.

There were varied amounts of relief experienced by patients with all these interventions, with some being more effective than others. The neuromodulation techniques mentioned in the following will show that neuromodulation is having a significant impact as a treatment option for fibromyalgia patients. Using current studies and analyzing the results, there is an overwhelming amount of evidence that proves the intervention of neuromodulation is beneficial to treating fibromyalgia[3].

Management by devices
Invasive neuromodulation
Spinal cord stimulation

Spinal cord stimulation has been around since 1967, when it was first introduced by Dr. Norman Shealy. It is currently used for a wide variety of chronic conditions in pain management with great success.

One study of note is an 11-year retrospective cohort study performed at the Mayo Clinic. Two cohorts of patients, one of individuals diagnosed with fibromyalgia and the other without. The outcomes in pain management for these two groups were monitored for 11 years with exposure to spinal cord stimulation. Patients in this study were asked to report their pain at 6 and 12 months after implantation of the spinal cord stimulator. At 6 months, patients in the fibromyalgia group reported a mean percentage change in pain of 46% less pain. In the group without fibromyalgia, the mean percentage change in pain was 50.9% less pain.

At the 12-month mark, patients with fibromyalgia reported an average percentage change in pain of about 43% less pain. On the other hand, the group with fibromyalgia reported an average percentage change in pain of about 47.9% less pain[5].

Spinal cord stimulation is proven to help provide pain relief to those with fibromyalgia. According to this study, patients with fibromyalgia can expect to achieve the same amount of pain relief as those without fibromyalgia. Spinal cord stimulation is certainly a plausible method to provide pain relief to those with fibromyalgia as individuals see their pain lessen, as well as not having to take as many opioids[5]. Patient selection is key to providing good outcomes, spinal cord stimulation will not work for all patients with fibromyalgia, and it covers pain in certain parts of the body only.

Deep brain stimulation

Deep brain stimulation (DBS) involves the implementation of electrodes into specific subcortical regions to produce an electric current. This method has been well tolerated by patients and carries low risk, like the other neuromodulation techniques discussed in this chapter. It is important to note that DBS clinical studies that were conducted did not meet efficacy criteria and thus did not receive FDA approval. This pursuit of FDA approval was not continued, and thus, DBS in the context of pain management and fibromyalgia is not supported by medical insurance reimbursement. Therefore, DBS is not widely used to treat fibromyalgia or chronic pain in general.

Deep brain stimulation has been used as a chronic pain treatment option since the 1970s, but the indications for situations that would warrant DBS are still not completely agreed upon.
However, there have been some positive results in treating certain pain conditions such as post-stroke pain, phantom limb syndrome, brachial

plexus injury, etc. As of now, DBS is not a clear solution to chronic pain conditions, with the results not sufficient to deem it a viable option. A meta-analysis conducted by Dr. Nour Shaheen over the current state of DBS shows that DBS has beneficial implications for chronic pain management. There is currently strong evidence that suggests it is a great option for facial neuropathic pain and traumatic subgroup pain subgroups. Further testing and research need to be done, along with FDA approval, for this method to progress to the level of being a viable option for fibromyalgia and other chronic pain conditions[6].

Intrathecal pump

An intrathecal pump, also commonly known as a pain pump, is a device implanted into the body that provides medication directly to the spinal cord and nerves. This device consists of a pump and reservoir placed in the abdomen and a catheter placed in the intrathecal space of the spinal cord[7].

Right now, interventional pain management physicians who use the intrathecal pain pump will first determine if the pain pump is the best option for the patient. Then, if the pain pump is deemed a good fit, a trial pump will be placed in the individual to see if there is any pain relief before moving forward. There are a few different types of trial pumps that the physician may recommend. The physician may recommend an injection, a series of injections, or a continuous trial. For the continuous trial, the device would be outside of your body for easy access and removal, if necessary, when assessed after trial completion. If the trial goes well, the pain pump will be implanted permanently and under your skin[4].

Intrathecal pumps can be used to treat fibromyalgia and have been shown to provide great pain relief to the right individual. A case study was conducted on a 44-year-old female who suffered from severe fibromyalgia pain. She had an opioid tolerance and had significant side effects from other medication options. The intrathecal pump was giving her 10 to 20 mg of morphine for 5 days and then switched to a 3 to 4 mg morphine-sulfate infusion. Over three months, the individual saw great decreases in her pain as well as disruptions to her sleep. The intrathecal pump is a great option for individuals suffering from refractory fibromyalgia[8].

Non-invasive neuromodulation

Quell Fibromyalgia (TENS)

Transcutaneous electrical nerve stimulation (TENS) is the delivery of pulsed electrical currents across the skin to stimulate peripheral nerves. TENS is a cheaper neuromodulation method that can also be self-administered[9].

A study conducted to see the effectiveness of two simultaneously active TENS devices on fibromyalgia pain was conducted. Currently, the use of one TENS device is a proven modality for aiding fibromyalgia pain. However, there has been limited research done using multiple TENS devices. This study had a placebo group, a single tens group, and a double tens group. The experimental groups had two TENS devices working but at different positions on the individual. The three positions were the lower back (5th lumbar vertebrae), above the C7 and T1 space, and below the C7 and T1 space[11].

The mean VAS pain score of the individuals during the duration of the study is displayed in the figure above. As shown in the line graph, the double tens line shows the most significant drop in pain score when compared to the single tens group and the placebo group. This study also shows that from a medication standpoint, the double tens group was using less and less pain medication, also showing the double tens method is more effective at pain reduction[11].

There is also currently a device out on the market called Quell Fibromyalgia. This is a wearable TENS device that can be controlled through an app on your phone. The Quell device is a disposable electrode inside of a small band that is wrapped around your upper calf. After the device is active, then the device will be linked to your phone, where you can view all of your data and health insights. This can be used for monitoring your health easily and at your discretion. Quell Fibromyalgia is currently the only FDA-approved medical device that helps with reducing the symptoms of Fibromyalgia. It is important to note that to acquire this device, you must have it prescribed, and it cannot be purchased on your own[12].

Transcranial direct current stimulation (tDCS)

Transcranial direct current stimulation (tDCS) uses small, constant currents, 1-2 mA) to modulate brain activity. Well known for its affordability and tolerance, tDCS is a prominent non-invasive neuromodulation method. A notable difference between TMS and tDCS is that TMS stimulates neuronal firing with suprathreshold stimulation, while tDCS polarizes the resting membrane potential.

The use of cathodal transcranial direct current stimulation (c-tDCS) on the S1, M1, and DLPFC parts of the brain has been shown to reduce fibromyalgia pain through reduction of hyperexcitable of the brain. This has also been shown to increase pain threshold and reduce sensitivity. Several studies have long debated whether anodal transcranial direct current stimulation (a-tDCS) is better than c-tDCS for certain parts of the brain. These studies also debate over which method targeting certain regions of the brain provides the best management of fibromyalgia symptoms, as well as adding to the longstanding contest over which version of transcranial direct current stimulation is the best[10].

One study that was performed tested the benefits of tDCS on females who were diagnosed with fibromyalgia. The goal of this study was to determine whether ten sessions of tDCS would be beneficial to treating fibromyalgia. The three experimental groups were a sham group, a tDCS group that targeted the M1 region, and a tDCS group that targeted another region of the brain called the DLPFC. Subjects would then follow up 30 and 60 days after the last session was administered, and their VAS scores would be recorded. The results were that the M1 group experienced significant pain relief that lasted past the 60-day mark. However, the DLPFC also had significant pain relief, but the relief only lasted for a short period.

In addition, quality of life was assessed using a Fibromyalgia impact questionnaire. This questionnaire asked the individuals in this study to assess their quality of life about function, fatigue, sleep disturbance, and psychological stress. Although all groups experienced some form of improved quality of life, only the M1 group experienced a statistically significant improvement. Overall, tDCS is a great treatment option for fibromyalgia patients, specifically for the M1 regions, for the best results[13].

Electroconvulsive therapy

Electroconvulsive therapy (ECT) involves applying an electric potential to the brain using electrodes. These electrodes will be affixed to the scalp and create electric fields. In one study conducted by (Usui et al. 2006), they tracked regional cerebral blood flow (rCBF) in individuals before and after ECT. The results showed that there was an increase in blood flow in the thalamic region, correlating with reduced pain scores in individuals.

Neurological imaging supports this study as the prefrontal cortex, anterior cingulate cortex, insula, and amygdala have been shown to have abnormal amounts of blood flow in chronic pain individuals. ECT, therefore, can help with fibromyalgia as it can restabilize the blood flow levels, which in turn provides pain relief[10].

Overall, this ECT study is the first of its kind to show that ECT is potentially a viable option for fibromyalgia patients who do not have a history of depression. The study shows that there were little to no changes in the patient's mood scores before and after ECT, thus showing that ECT operates independently of mood and can now be used on individuals without depression for treatment[16]. The decrease in thalamic blood flow that is solved by ECT treatment is the main takeaway, with mood improvements being minimal, patients with fibromyalgia not presenting with depression or a history of depression could use ECT[16].

Electroconvulsive therapy has shown that it can target fibromyalgia symptoms without having too much of an impact on a patient's mood, which is a great finding. This allows this treatment to be more commonly used as it has the application to be used on a greater number of patients without causing serious adverse risks when affecting moods. The next step is to have more studies on a larger scale using electroconvulsive therapy to see if the results hold up when using a larger sample size.

Transcranial alternating current stimulation (tACS)

Transcranial alternating current stimulation (tACS) involves a sinusoidal alternating current to the scalp, also generating an electric field. Like transcranial direct current stimulation (tDCS), both methods affect cortical excitability. Transcranial alternating current stimulation is more precise in directing endogenous brain oscillations. This method is better at mimicking our natural brain oscillations and, thus, more effective at regulating the brain.

In one study, tACS was used on patients with fibromyalgia in a series of 10 20-minute stimulation sessions. This was applied to the left part of the M1 region of the brain. When comparing the results between the experimental group and the sham, the results showed that there was a positive result. Patients reported less overall pain. However, there was not enough of a difference to deem it statistically significant[17].

Transcranial alternating current stimulation is a relatively newer method compared to others. However, there have been promising results with innovative tACS techniques and overall advancement. This serves as a promising avenue for fibromyalgia treatment in the future with further testing[10].

Transcranial random noise stimulation (tRNS)

Transcranial random noise stimulation (tRNS) differs from the other transcranial stimulation techniques due to the lower discomfort levels experienced by patients. In an analgesic study, tRNS showed that it can provide not only immediate but also long-lasting effects. The benefits were seen when applied to the m1 area of the cerebral cortex. As a newer and less known method of neuromodulation, tRNS displays the potential for long-term pain reduction through neuroplasticity[10].

In one study that tested motor cortex tRNS as an effective treatment not only for fibromyalgia pain but also for cognitive and mood effects, the results were great. This study was conducted by recruiting 20 female patients with a fibromyalgia diagnosis. The patients in this study were subjected to tRNS 5 times a week for two weeks, with their results recorded. The results for whether the tRNS were recorded after the two weeks of the study. Overall, the results show that the patient's overall pain scores and the impact of fibromyalgia on their lives decreased by a significant amount throughout the study.

The patients also described themselves as feeling more active. Additionally, HADS scores were recorded, which show the impact on mood. There was a significantly significant decrease as well, which shows there was an improvement in mood. This includes improved anxiety and decreased depression symptoms. The tRNS also improved the "fibrofog" cognitive dysfunction frequently associated with fibromyalgia. Lastly, tRNS was safe and well tolerated by the patients. Only one patient reported a slight "hot" sensation during the duration of the experiment[18].

Reduced impedance non-invasive cortical electrostimulation (RINCE)

Reduced impedance non-invasive cortical electrostimulation (RINCE) is also a newer and unexplored method. In RINCE, the electrodes are attached to the patient's scalp but generate a specific frequency. This allows the current to enter deeper into the cerebral cortex by lowering the impedance of the skin and skull. This could lead to better results with pain reduction. However, there are minimal results out there to support or negate this method. In one study conducted, the RINCE method was shown to improve the pain threshold in a fibromyalgia treatment group when compared to a sham group. Additionally, the fibromyalgia patients reported lower pain scores after the RINCE treatment[10].

There have been some mild side effects, including headache, nausea, dizziness, vertigo, and localized skin reactions. However, these side effects were short-lived, and on average, only two of the listed effects were experienced by a patient[15].

These results are promising as the difference between the fibromyalgia and the sham group is statistically significant. More research and studies need to be conducted. However, there is optimism surrounding the RINSE method[10].

Transcranial magnetic stimulation (TMS)

Transcranial magnetic stimulation is a technique in which an inductor and a capacitor generate changing magnetic fields. The reverse current that is produced as a result of this changing magnetic field thus affects specific regions of the brain, neuronal functions, and overall electrical activity. The threshold for determining the stimulation intensity ranges from 80 to 120% of the individual's resting motor threshold.

Fibromyalgia patients found some success with transcranial magnetic stimulation (TMS). After about ten sessions of TMS, fibromyalgia patients experienced significant pain relief. In comparison to pharmacological methods, TMS is safer, with individuals showing fewer side effects. Additionally, TMS has been shown to also target other fibromyalgia symptoms such as sleep disruptions, functional impairments, as well as overall fatigue[10].

As of right now, there have been three studies performed that dive into TMS being used in patients with fibromyalgia. One study looked into the use of TMS in treating patients with treatment-resistant depression and borderline personality disorder, with 4 of the subjects having been diagnosed with fibromyalgia. Throughout the study, the experimental groups varied in the amount of TMS they were receiving through intervals of strength of the electrical stimulation.

Overall, all groups experienced some form of pain relief from their fibromyalgia, with some individuals even feeling 100% relief. The patients were contacted after the study to see how long their pain relief was sustained around 15-27 weeks after the conclusion of the study was the timeframe (Sampson 2006). The stimulation was applied to the R-DLPFC region of the brain and shows prefrontal cortical stimulation can be a viable option for fibromyalgia patients[14].

The second study also used a similar experimental design as the previously mentioned experiment. However, there was also more randomization and a placebo. Also of note, this study was done on a much larger scale. The results show that there was not too much of a difference in pain relief, although there was some (Graff-Guerero 2005). However, these individuals were subjected to much smaller doses, which could be the cause of the results being less pronounced[14].

Lastly, the third study was done similarly, except all individuals were subjected to the same level of electrical stimulation. The level of stimulation was a 25 series of 8-second pulse trains with 52-second intervals between series. This was at a 10 Hz and 80% resting motor threshold frequency. The outcome of this study would be determined through an eleven-point numerical scale and compared between groups through statistical analysis. Overall, this study shows that TMS of the primary motor cortex creates a long-lasting decrease in pain and improved quality of life in patients with fibromyalgia. This is accomplished without affecting mood or anxiety levels. The analgesic effects of TMS differed for the sensory and affective dimensions of pain, with the affective dimension change lasting 15 days longer[14].

Transcranial focused ultrasound (tFUS)

Transcranial-focused ultrasound is another emerging non-invasive neuromodulation technique that could be a possible option for fibromyalgia patients. Although this technique is not as well known or researched as some of the other methods discussed in this chapter, this technique has displayed incredible spatial precision with the ability to stimulate deep brain regions with millimeter accuracy[10].

When comparing tFUS to the current non-ultrasonic techniques such as tDCS, implanted electrode techniques, and TMS, transcranial ultrasonic neuromodulation offers a unique combination of high resolution in space (a few millimeters) and time (a few hundred milliseconds). This gives us great access to deep brain structures. tFUS neuromodulation could thus allow us to obtain high-resolution and non-invasive neuromodulation applications such as the treatment of fibromyalgia patients. There have been results completed in other studies that show tFUS has benefits in modulating the level of cortical neurotransmitters[19].

Overall, there needs to be further research and experimentation with this neuromodulation technique to confirm the current results of benefits. More studies using this technique on a larger sample size should be conducted to have more reliable results.

References:

1. "Interventional Pain Management for Fibromyalgia." *Momentum Medical*, 31 July 2023, momentuminjury.com/interventional-pain-management-for-fibromyalgia/.
2. Clauw, Daniel, et al. "The Science of Fibromyalgia." *Mayo Clinic Proceedings*, Elsevier, 23 Dec. 2011, www.sciencedirect.com/science/article/pii/S0025619611652233?casa_token=bDaD0A5zK9QAAAAA%3A_6iFlGGd0eiOy0SmtrMrMmC54YZ-_BbVaxgXfp87fbnc0z4icYLjnU7XaIBQyd5CiywiKhxQQII.
3. Cheng, Ying-Cheh. "Treating Fibromyalgia with Electrical Neuromodulation: A Systematic Review and Meta-Analysis." *Clinical Neurophysiology*, Elsevier, 1 Feb. 2023, www.sciencedirect.com/science/article/pii/S1388245723000202?via%3Dihub.
4. "Do I Need a Pain Pump?" *Interventional Pain Center*, 2 Apr. 2024, columbuspain.com/do-i-need-a-pain-pump/#:~:text=Sachida%20Manocha%2C%20MD%2C%20of%20Interventional,pain%2C%20neuropathy%2C%20and%20fibromyalgia.
5. D'Souza, Ryan. "Does Fibromyalgia Affect the Outcomes of Spinal Cord Stimulation: An 11-Year, Multicenter, Retrospective Matched Cohort Study." *Neuromodulation: Technology at the Neural Interface*, Elsevier, 13 July 2022, www.sciencedirect.com/science/article/pii/S1094715922007231?casa_token=vwRpqPAJ6sQAAAAA%3ALzvKPcb9umKyw

xZYalfH45glYrOmumdDDwrOQXcIcuea3LyIPGUvU5mdE11laisnXkuPYQLC5Q.

6. Shaheen, Nour, et al. "Deep brain stimulation for chronic pain: a systematic review and meta-analysis." *Frontiers in human neuroscience* vol. 17 1297894. 30 Nov. 2023, doi:10.3389/fnhum.2023.1297894

7. "Intrathecal Pain Pump." *Johns Hopkins Medicine*, 7 Apr. 2023, www.hopkinsmedicine.org/health/treatment-tests-and-therapies/intrathecal-pain-pump.

8. Ju, Yu Mi, et al. "Implantable Drug Delivery Systems with Morphine in Fibromyalgia -a Case Report-." *Anesthesia and Pain Medicine*, The Korean Society of Anesthesiologists, 31 Jan. 2017, synapse.koreamed.org/articles/1158286.

9. Johnson, Mark. "Transcutaneous Electrical Nerve Stimulation (TENS) for Fibromyalgia In Adults" *Cochrane Library*, 9 Oct. 2017, www.cochranelibrary.com/cdsr/doi/10.1002/14651858.CD012172.pub2/full.

10. Zhang, Jia-Hao, et al. "Non-invasive brain stimulation for fibromyalgia: current trends and future perspectives." *Frontiers in neuroscience* vol. 17 1288765. 19 Oct. 2023, doi:10.3389/fnins.2023.1288765

11. Lauretti, Gabriela, et al. "Efficacy of the Use of Two Simultaneously Tens Devices for Fibromyalgia Pain - Rheumatology International." *SpringerLink*, Springer Berlin Heidelberg, 20 Feb. 2013, link.springer.com/article/10.1007/s00296-013-2699-y.

12. Quell Fibromylagia. "For Physicians." *Quell Fibromyalgia*, 2 Jan. 2024, quellfibromyalgia.com/for-physicians/.
13. Valle, Angela, et al. "Efficacy of anodal transcranial direct current stimulation (tDCS) for the treatment of fibromyalgia: results of a randomized, sham-controlled longitudinal clinical trial." *Journal of pain management* vol. 2,3 (2009): 353-361.
14. Short, Baron et al. "Non-invasive brain stimulation approaches to fibromyalgia pain." *Journal of pain management* vol. 2,3 (2009): 259-276.
15. Szymoniuk, Michał. "Brain Stimulation for Chronic Pain Management: A Narrative Review of Analgesic Mechanisms and Clinical Evidence - Neurosurgical Review." *SpringerLink*, Springer Berlin Heidelberg, 29 May 2023, link.springer.com/article/10.1007/s10143-023-02032-1#Sec3.
16. Usui, Chie. "Electroconvulsive Therapy Improves Severe Pain Associated with Fibromyalgia." *Pain*, Elsevier, 21 Feb. 2006, www.sciencedirect.com/science/article/abs/pii/S0304395906000029.
17. Lin, Ashleigh Peng, et al. "Using High-Definition Transcranial Alternating Current Stimulation to Treat Patients with Fibromyalgia: A Randomized Double-Blinded Controlled Study." *MDPI*, Multidisciplinary Digital Publishing Institute, 31 Aug. 2022, www.mdpi.com/2075-1729/12/9/1364.
18. Curatolo, M. "Motor Cortex tRNS Improves Pain, Affective and Cognitive Impairment in Patients with Fibromyalgia: Preliminary Results of a Randomised Sham-Controlled Trial." *Clinical and Experimental Rheumatology*, 2017,

file:///Users/milanpatel/Downloads/article.pdf.
19. Aubry, Jean-François. "MR-Guided Transcranial Focused Ultrasound." *SpringerLink*, Springer International Publishing, 1 Jan. 2016, link.springer.com/chapter/10.1007/978-3-319-22536-4_6.

Notes

www.ingramcontent.com/pod-product-compliance
Lightning Source LLC
Chambersburg PA
CBHW031627210526
45464CB00004B/1781